ketoCONTINUUM
Workbook

ketoCONTINUUM

Workbook

The Steps to be Consistently Keto for Life

Annette Bosworth, M.D.

Dr. Boz®

MEDICAL DISCLAIMER

The information presented in this book is the result of years of practice experience. The information in this book is general in nature and not a substitute for an evaluation and advice by a competent medical specialist. The content provided is for educational purposes and does not take the place of the doctor-patient relationship. Every effort has been made to ensure that the content provided is accurate, helpful and understandable. However, this is not an exhaustive coverage of the subject. No liability is assumed. You are responsible for your own health.

ketoCONTINUUM Workbook
The Steps to be Consistently Keto for Life

By

Annette Bosworth, MD

ISBN-13 Digits: 978-1-7361661-2-3

MeTone Life, LLC

ISBN-10 Digits: 1-7361661-2-3

Published in the United States by MeTone Life, LLC

3204 Madelyn Ave, Sioux Falls, SD 57106

ketoCONTINUUM Workbook

About the Author   viii

Why A Workbook   ix

1

Before You Begin   1
1.1   Write Down Your Why   2
1.2   Form Your Tribe   10
1.3   Supplies & Measurements   12
1.4   Cupboard Therapy   28
1.5   Trouble Clubs   30

2

Keto First Week   32
2.1.   Day 1: Begin   33
2.2   Day 2: Eat Fat   35
2.3   Day 3: Pray for Pink   39
2.4   Day 4: Oh Poop!   41
2.5   No Ketones: End of Day 4   49
2.6   Setbacks & Stalls   55
2.7   Day 5: Magnesium   57
2.8   Day 6: Calories & Cravings   62
2.9   Meetings & Mirror Neurons   77

3

Becoming Keto Adapted   85
3.1   Week 2 Challenges   86
3.2   ketoCONTINUUM #3   94
3.3   ketoCONTINUUM #4   98

4

Baseline Metabolism — 102

4.1 Overview of Baseline Metabolisms — 103

4.2 ketoCONTINUUM #5 — 107

4.3 Measuring Ketones & Dr Boz Ratio — 113

4.4 ketoCONTINUUM #6 — 125

4.5 ketoCONTINUUM #7 — 129

4.6 ketoCONTINUUM #8 — 135

5

Fasting Cycles — 143

5.1 Overview of Fasting Cycles — 144

5.2 ketoCONTINUUM #9 & #10 — 152

5.3 ketoCONTINUUM #11 & 12 — 162

COMPILED RESOURCES — 184

Links Throughout the Book — 185

Charts — 187

ABOUT THE AUTHOR

Annette Bosworth, MD, (Dr. Boz), is an internal medicine physician, and a leading authority in optimizing brain health. Author of the runaway bestseller, *Anyway You Can*: A Beginner's Guide to Ketones for Life, has helped patients overcome long-term chronic conditions such as obesity, depression, autoimmune problems, and addiction. She accomplishes all of this by applying lifestyle adjustments, teaching preventive medicine, and other practical medical interventions.

Dr. Boz is a frequent lecturer at youth shelters, schools, universities, churches, jails, leadership seminars, and the military. Through the Department of Defense and Counter-terrorism agencies, she loves teaching the nation's front-line defenders how to optimize their brains and bodies with applicable neuroscience.

In addition to running her private medical clinic, Dr. Boz has taught at the University Of Utah and University of South Dakota School Of Medicines. Teaching health and wellness has been a recurring theme in Dr. Boz's career. Born into a farming family in rural South Dakota, she witnessed first-hand the importance of each individual's contribution to strengthening a community. Dr. Boz's Internal Medicine practice intimately works with her patients, refusing to give up on them when others, and sometimes the patients have. Dr. Boz strives to deliver "Meaningful Medicine" one ketone at a time.

Dr. Boz's steadfast desire for first-class patient care hasn't gone unnoticed. She has been featured on CNN, Time Magazine, US News & World Report, Fox News, and other major news outlets. Despite her rigorous schedule, Dr. Boz leads volunteer medical mission trips to Haiti, the Philippines, and many underserved communities in her home state of South Dakota.

Along with her husband, Dr. Boz savors the adventure of raising three energetic, fast-growing sons through debate, wrestling, music, and theater in Sioux Falls, South Dakota.

Contact Dr. Boz: www.BozMD.com

WHY A WORKBOOK

ANYWAY YOU CAN

In my first book, ANYWAY YOU CAN, I shared the story of Grandma Rose, my mom. Her relief from cancer through keto-chemistry swept through readers around the world. The book became a sensation and emerged as one of the best keto books for explaining ketone nutrition. Why?

Is it because the writing was perfect? No. Is it because I had every fact about keto figured out? Certainly not.

ANYWAY YOU CAN shared a true love story. My dying mother needed a teacher and a friend. God blessed me with the skills to answer her needs. Something deep in my soul mandated me to slow down and help her. Grandma Rose stood on the edge of her grave. I took her hand and coaxed her away from the edge with loving lessons about ketogenic nutrition. ANYWAY YOU CAN exposed my skepticism of this whacky approach. It shared my fears and insecurities along with the keto-lessons I taught Grandma Rose. By the grace of God, it worked. Her health improved along with my knowledge of this strange diet. The story inspired readers to use ketogenic nutrition, ANYWAY YOU CAN.

This workbook along with the teachings from my second book ketoCONTINUUM take my instructions of keto-chemistry to the next level.

WHY A WORKBOOK.

Think back to the last time life got stressful. You know that habit that you thought you'd kicked? But in a moment of stress, the kicked-habit invaded your mind again.

You'd given up smoking years ago. Yet, when you lost your job or your friend died, thoughts of cigarettes flooded your mind. They flashed through your private fortress without your permission. Betraying you.

You vowed not to partake in the office gossip. Yet, last week a time of boredom pulled you in as someone shared a story that wasn't theirs to tell.

What made you think of that cigarette? What made you lean in?

Those old habits are hard to break. Change requires support. A tribe. A group.

At age 71, Grandma Rose beat the odds. Longstanding change did not happen because her daughter was a doctor. Switching to keto-nutrition was the easy part. Along with the instructions of "How To," Grandma Rose needed the support that encircled her and kept her accountable.

This workbook offers the steps needed to start, the roadmap of where you are going, and the charts to master your ketoCONTINUUM.

"DR BOZ, HOW DO I DO THIS? EXACTLY."

This workbook answers this question.

When ANYWAY YOU CAN was published, I told many of my internal medicine patients to, "Read at least the first five chapters before coming back."

Through Grandma Rose's story, the information trickled into their minds. Further curiosity attracted them to our local support group, where I answered their questions. They saw real examples of how to apply this change of health. This process worked better than many of my prescriptions.

Folks outside my practice area struggled with the exact steps to take.

This workbook is the HOW TO manual for consistently staying keto.

If you started the ketogenic diet and fell off, this workbook is for you.

If you read Grandma Rose's story and had intentions of doing the ketogenic diet but never quite got there, this workbook is for you.

If you watched YouTube lectures and wanted to try this but didn't know how to start, this workbook is for you.

If you have tried time-restricted eating or fasting but could not stick to the rhythm, this workbook is for you.

If you have co-workers that want to do the ketogenic diet but don't know how to begin, this workbook is perfect.

Let me help you.

This workbook takes you through the steps I use to help patients.

HELP YOUR DOCTOR HELP YOU.

How do doctors manage a patient on ketogenic nutrition? Often, they don't.

It took me the better part of a year to fit keto into my medical practice. Most doctors will not take that time. Help your doctor.

Use this workbook and take it to your next appointment.

HELPFUL TIPS FOR USING THIS WORKBOOK

This workbook sets up successful change for a lifetime. You may have tried keto in the past. Maybe you succeeded at first and then stopped seeing improvement. This workbook will guide you with the tools needed to obtain your best health.

If you have never tried keto, start from the beginning and proceed sequentially.

The charts throughout the book fit a season of change. If you struggle with a particular section, use the coordinated chart to navigate out of the rut and into a successful rhythm.

Notice the header in the upper corner of the right-sided pages in the workbook. The chapter of the book ketoCONTINUUM that correlates to the section is noted there. Refer to those sections of the book if you want more information about the instructions.

Section 1 prepares you for sustainable change. In addition, you will find tips for those who failed their first attempt.

Section 2 steps you through the first seven days of keto nutrition. Next, section 3 coaches you into keto adaption while helping you settle into ketoCONTINUUM #3 & #4.

Sections 4 and 5 map out the long game. I am particularly fond of the charts in these final sections. They are designed to help you recognize patterns.

Use these charts. The charts offer tiny adjustments when you compare them to one another. These small steps corrected massive metabolism issues in many of my patients. They achieved optimal results when they held a newly changed behavior until they perfected the habit. The charts will help you study yourself. You will find patterns of behavior when reflecting on the charts after you've filled in several lines.

ROADMAP

The chart ketoCONTINUUM roadmaps the plan to stay consistently keto. The chart outlines where you are going and where you've been.

Don't study this now.

Gently glance over the far left column. You will start out as a beginner and eventually move to baseline metabolisms. The far-right column estimates the time to get there.

ketoCONTINUUMS #5 through #8 are where you should strive to live.

To achieve your best health, you may or may not need to stress your metabolism. ketoCONTINUUMs #9 through #12 offer workouts for your metabolism. Use these options intermittently to help inch toward your optimum health.

ketoCONTINUUM ROADMAP

	ketoCONTINUUM	WHO DOES THE WORK?	TEST	GUIDELINES	NEXT STEPS	
BEGINNER	**#1:** I eat every 2–4 hours	CHEMISTRY CARRIES YOU	X	Fueled on glucose. Must refuel often. Never fueled by ketones.		4–6 WEEKS
	#2: I eat every 6–8 hours LESS THAN 20 total carbs		Urine PeeTone Strips	Eat <20 total carbs per day. Ketosis begins. Fat-based hormones rise. Eating happens less frequently.	Be sure to eat high fat with low carbs. Your body uses the fat to restore your fat built hormones. Elevated insulin within your body prevents you from using the stored fat. You must eat the fat.	
	#3: I "accidentally" missed a meal. [Keto-adapted]			Fat supplies the resources needed to make fat-built hormones approach healthy levels. Appetite decreases according to body's chemistry.	Sometimes it takes 10 weeks before this moment happens. Don't look at the scale. Listen for absence of hunger.	
	#4: Eat 2 meals per day	YOU DO THE WORK. Discipline needed for each new step.		Choose to eat only 2 meals per day.	Succeed 7 days in a row before advancing.	
BASELINE METABOLISM	**#5:** 16:8			Eat ALL food, snacks and supplements in an 8-hour window. No eating, snacking or chewing for 16 hours.	That means no gum during fasting hours. Suck on salt if you need a substitute. Keep your coffee filled with fat.	LIVE HERE
	#6: Advanced 16:8			Clean up your morning drink. Remove all calories and sweeteners. Morning drink = no fat, no MCT, no butter, no sweeteners, no calories. The 16 hours = only salt, water, black coffee or tea.	Don't remove the fat from your morning drink before this phase. You needed it to get here. Now it's time to let it go.	
	#7: 23:1 OMAD ALL in one hour			ALL calories and sweeteners in one hour. 23 hours = Only salt, water, tea or coffee.	Begin checking blood numbers right before you eat.	
	#8: Advanced 23:1/OMAD	PSYCHOLOGY. Use tribe for best results.	Blood Ketone Strips	Move eating-hour within 11 hours following sunrise to match your circadian rhythm.	Record the Dr. Boz ratio first thing in the morning. Repeat before eating.	
STRESSING METABOLISM	**#9:** 36-hour fast			Fast for 36 hours. No calories. No sweeteners. Start in evening as to use 2 cycles of sleep during the 36 hours.	Begin fast after evening meal. DANGER: If on blood pressure meds or blood sugar lowing meds. ASK YOUR DOCTOR.	USE INTERMITTENTLY
	#10: 36-hour fast without a celebration meal			After 36-hour fast, return to your normal pattern of eating without a splurge meal.	Offer a group fasting routine to others in your tribe. Fast together.	
	#11: 48-hour fast			Fast for 48 hours. No calories. No sweeteners.	Safe to try twice a week. Unlike the 36-hour fast, this option keeps meals at the same time each day.	
	#12: 72-hour fast			Fast for 72 hours. No calories. No sweeteners.	When the timing is right, stress your metabolism with 8 weeks of a 72-hour fast. The rest of the week, return to your BASELINE METABOLISM. The best transitions happen through this challenge.	

Three Metabolic Stages:

Beginner:

ketoCONTINUUM #1 represents most menu-habits across the globe. This row offers a starting place on your journey. It also marks the landing place if you fall. Use the chart on the opposite page to date when you started changing your health and if you fall out of habit. This chart will show you a pattern over the next year. Use it.
Document the dates when you start each ketoCONTINUUM.

If you struggle to make a lasting transition into any of the ketoCONTINUUMs, document the dates you try again. Failing is part of everyone's education. Notice the success of how long you stay the course on the second or third attempt. Less time spent off the wagon is a WIN.

Graduate from Beginner to Baseline Metabolism when you choose to eat only two meals per day for a week.
ketoCONTINUUM #4 is the bridge between Beginners and Baseline Metabolism. Choosing to eat fewer times per day marks a mental shift in your approach to ketogenic nutrition. Don't advance to #5 until you genuinely master ketoCONTINUUM #4.
The solid mastery of ketoCONTINUUM #4 will protect you. When patients fall off the keto-wagon, this is where I hope they land.

ketoCONTINUUM #4 preserves much of your keto-chemistry. Land at #4 when you fall off the wagon.

Baseline Metabolism:

ketoCONTINUUMS #5-#8 step you through a progression that slowly builds your metabolism. Metabolic strength grows on all four of these stages. Strong metabolisms improve your immune system, restore brainpower, and strengthen your muscles.
Find the baseline ketoCONTINUUM that matches your season of life and stay there.

- The charts in section 4 help you progress within ketoCONTINUUMs #5 through #8.

- These metabolic chapters should be practiced and perfected.

- It is not mandatory for you to advance to the highest baseline metabolism.

- Use the charts in section 4 to promote your metabolism until you achieve your health goals.

STRESSING METABOLISM:

Reach for these challenges periodically. These stresses will strengthen your metabolism. In addition, they will help you move through the baseline metabolisms. For example, if you struggle to move from #5 to #6, add a weekly fast of 36 hours for eight weeks in a row.

Adding a fast to your baseline metabolism challenges your metabolism much like weight lifting challenges a runner. Don't start bench pressing twice your bodyweight. Don't start with a 72-hour fast.

Learning to say, "NO" to food is a skill. As this skill improves, stretch the time you go without food.

USE THIS CHART TO TRACK YOUR OVERALL PROGRESS.

ketoCONTINUUM	Date								
1. I eat every 2–4 hours									
2. LESS THAN 20 total carbs									
3. I "accidentally" missed a meal. [Keto-adapted]									
4. Eat 2 meals per day									
5. 16:8									
6. Advanced 16:8									
7. 23:1 OMAD ALL in one hour									
8. Advanced 23:1/OMAD									
9. 36-hour fast									
10. 36-hour fast without a celebration meal									
11. 48-hour fast									
12. 72-hour fast									

ketoCONTINUUM

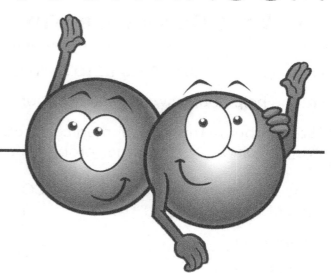

SECTION

1

BEFORE YOU BEGIN

1.1   Write Down Your Why

1.2   Form Your Tribe

1.3   Supplies & Measurements

1.4   Cupboard Therapy

1.5   Trouble Clubs

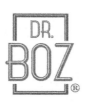

BozMD.com

1.1 WRITE DOWN YOUR WHY

WHY DO YOU WANT TO GO KETO? WHAT MOTIVATES YOU?

Let me help you answer these questions.

Read through this list of medical problems. Circle the items that have caused you to struggle or worry. Add other problems that have stolen your health.

- Too Heavy
  (want to lose weight)
- Joint Pain
- Inflammation
- Seizures
- Low Energy
- Cancer
- Multiple Sclerosis
- Fragile Immune System
- Autoimmune Problems
- Thyroid Problems
- Lupus
- Crohn's Disease
- Inflammatory Bowel
  Disease
- Heart Disease
- Irritable Bowel
- ADHD
- Depression
- Anxiety
- Infertility

- PCOS
- Acne/Desire Better Skin
- Alcoholism Addiction
- Brain Fog
- Diabetes
- High Blood Pressure
- Alzheimer's Disease
- Swollen Ankles
- Rotten Sleep

Medical problems are not a strong enough WHY to sustain the changes for a ketogenic diet. However, medical issues offer a starting place to find your WHY.

Mentally play forward what your life will look like if the medical problems don't improve. Write down what you will miss out on because of these medical issues.

_____

_____

_____

_____

_____

_____

_____

_____

_____

_____

_____

_____

_____

_____

_____

_____

_____

_____

Take a deep breath. Let it out slowly. After reading the following sentence, close your eyes and imagine this moment.

Think of the best moment of your life.
Please think of the day when joy, acceptance, attraction, or love flowed through your soul. Mothers, don't be tricked into a "correct" answer like the day you gave birth to a child. That was a tough day. It can be the days following childbirth if you can find a specific memory. You will know you have found the answer when you feel an emotion as you think of the moment. You get goosebumps. You feel tears begin to form as you think of that time. You can often picture the people that joined you in that moment very clearly.

If several moments come to your mind, find the one that created the most intense emotion.

Without the restoration of your health, moments like this will be missed. This is an example of a WHY. Write down your moment.

_____

_____

_____

_____

_____

_____

_____

_____

_____

_____

_____

_____

Now turn your perspective the other direction. Think back to the worst moment of your life—a time where the world disappointed you. Life was cruel, and no hero showed up to the rescue. You were hurt. Embarrassed. Shamed. Alone and without support.

Document that moment. Write it down.
Don't be cheap about this exercise. Reach for the story that hurts —the one that changed the trajectory of your childhood.

How does that story impact your life today? Does it relate to the way you comfort yourself? Weave the pain of this moment into your WHY.

_____

_____

_____

_____

_____

_____

_____

_____

_____

_____

_____

_____

_____

_____

As you crystalized that moment from your past, think about the people that helped make that moment happen. Think about the people that meant the most to you as you traveled through your childhood. Even if they were not present for that most significant moment of your life, recognize how their influence created part of your personality. Then, write down those people and the role they played in your life.

ketoCONTINUUM Workbook

Now think about repeating that peak moment in your life. Write down a dream for your future where you could live out the repeat of the best moment of your life. Be sure to mention with whom you would share that moment. This time consider sharing it with someone you love. Maybe you're receiving the attention and affection, or perhaps you are offering that gift to someone else.

Once the stories from the previous pages have been documented, leave this section alone for a day or two.

When you return to this project, look over your entries. The previous pages hold your WHY. You will know you have found it when you reread the section and it evokes the most potent emotion—circle that section.

Summarize your why here:

_____

_____

_____

_____

_____

_____

_____

_____

_____

_____

_____

_____

_____

_____

_____

_____

ketoCONTINUUM **Workbook**

1.2 FORM YOUR TRIBE

STEPS TO FORM YOUR GROUP

WRITE THIS SIGNUP:

Write down these words: "I am starting a keto support group to improve my health. Join me, please. Every Tuesday at 3:30 - 4:30 PM in the conference room. Starts in August. Will continue through October and then re-assess. Please come."

Handwritten signs work better than printed ones. Consider adding tear-offs along the bottom with the time and address. Notice your commitment lasts for three months. Once this sign-up hangs on a wall for others to read, you have accountability.

WHO

Focus on attracting people, not the location.
Write down five places you interact with people. (examples: office, church, the kids' school activities, and volunteer groups).

1. _____   4. _____

2. _____   5. _____

3. _____

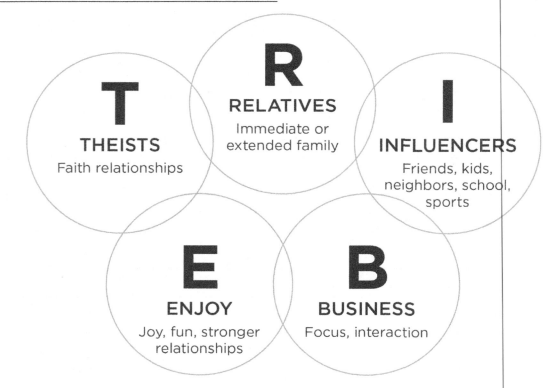

Next, write down five people that you could reach out to in a moment of struggle. When tragedy or sadness hits your life, who would call? Write down their names.

1. _____

2. _____

3. _____

4. _____

5. _____

POST SIGNUP AT YOUR 5 LOCATIONS. HAND THE SIGNUP TO YOUR 5 PEOPLE.

FOR NOW, that's all I want you to do for your support group. Section 2.9 finishes this thought process.

IN 2.9, WE WILL COVER THE FOLLOWING DETAILS.

- Location of meeting
- Frequency of meeting
- Cost of meeting
- Best Practices for a successful meeting
- The key rule about food
- Purpose of meetings
- Meeting curriculum

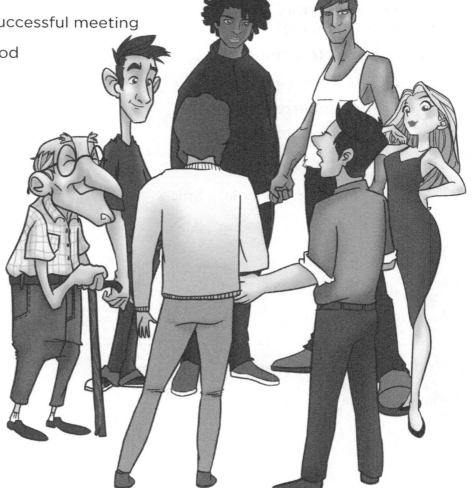

1.3 SUPPLIES & MEASUREMENTS

DON'T GROCERY SHOP YET.

Do not start with grocery shopping. Rushing towards the grocery store puts your focus in the wrong area. Instead, read through this list of supplies.

Buy the MUST-HAVES, consider buying the SHOULD HAVES, and read the few warnings.

MUST HAVES:

- A dozen eggs
- PeeTone Strips
- Cronometer Application
- Dr. Boz Food Guide - found on www.BozMD.com

SHOULD HAVES:

- Beta-Hydroxybutyrate Powder (Exogenous Ketones)
  - Dr. Boz Keto Combo
  - BHB Ketones-In-A-Can
    - Raspberry Lemonade
    - Cucumber Lemon
    - Dutch Chocolate
    - Mexican Chocolate Spice

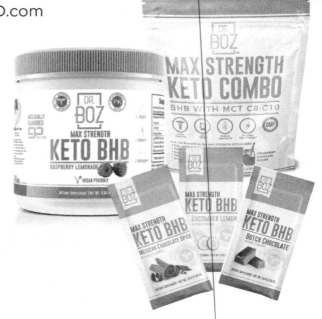

	Fats & Oils	Nuts & Seeds	Drinks/Alcohol	Sweets
Best	• C8:C10 MCT oil/powder (MCT = Medium Chain Triglycerides) Provides rapid, pure ketone production. • MCT oil/powder	• Pili nuts • Chia seeds • Macadamia nuts	• Water/Mineral water • Black coffee • Black tea/black chai tea • None (Alcohol STOPS ketone production.)	• None Sugar STOPS ketone production. Sugar substitutes slow ketone production way down.
Better	• Lard/Bacon grease • Mayonnaise • Butter • Avocado oil	• Pecans • Walnuts • Pumpkin seeds	• Coffee (with fat) • Tea (with fat) • Chai tea (with fat) • Distilled liquors	• Cinnamon • Dark chocolate (75% cacao or more)
Good	• Extra virgin olive oil • Coconut oil • Sesame oil • Grape seed oil	• Almonds • Hazelnuts • Peanuts	• Kombucha • Almond/Coconut milk • Red wine (very dry) • Carbohydrate free drinks (with sugar substitutes)	• Stevia • Monk fruit • Erythritol

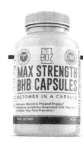

○Ketones-In-A-Capsule

○Medium Chain Triglycerides C8:C10 Oil

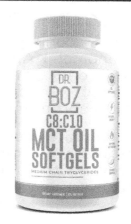

•Epsom Salt: Buy at least 15 pounds

   ▪ 5-pound bag= $12.00

   ▪ 50-pound bag= $40.00 You will use all of this.

• Milk of Magnesium: Unflavored. A generic version of this costs about $3.00. Buy it.

The rules of ketogenic nutrition are simple but odd. When compared to the standard American Diet groceries list, buying high fat, low carb is weird.

The Dr. Boz Keto Food Guide lists foods commonly eaten to achieve ketosis. The food guide sorts foods into good, better, and best choices. At first, reach for 'good' choices. Months from now, you will graduate to 'better' decisions. Ultimately, I encourage choosing the 'best' options as outlined in the guide.

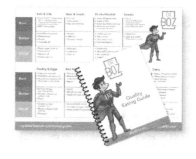

The guide displays the same information on a magnetic guide for the fridge and a pocket booklet. Take the booklet with you when shopping. If you have a kid (or a spouse) that wants to know what's allowed, say these words, "If it's not in that booklet, we don't buy it."

Within two short weeks, you'll look at a menu and know the dos and don'ts. Until then, use the guide. When you've mastered the information, pass it to someone else.

	Poultry & Eggs	Red Meat & Pork	Fish & Shellfish	Veggies & Fruits	Dairy
Best	• Eggs (yolk included) • Omelets (with added fat) • Homemade bone broth (should gel at room temp.)	• Ribs (braised) • Braunschweiger/Liverwurst • Bacon	• Mackerel • Herring • Albacore Tuna • Sardines • Salmon	• Spinach • Avocado • Kale • Cabbage (fermented or raw)	• Heavy whipping cream • Ghee (anhydrous butter) • Hard cheese (ex. parmesan)
Better	• Buffalo wings (with bleu cheese) • Chicken (with skin on, cooked in fat) • Duck	• Spam • Brisket (braised) • Marbled steak (with butter)	• Trout • Anchovies	• Brussels sprouts • Cauliflower • Green olives (fresh or in oil)	• Full fat cream cheese • Feta cheese • Bleu cheese • Sour cream
Good	• Chicken breast (cooked in fat) • Sliced turkey breast (add fat) • Pheasant	• Ground beef (full fat) • Sausage (no sugar added) • Hard salami/Pepperoni	• Cod • Oysters • Snapper • Shellfish	• Blackberries • Artichokes • Tomatoes • Rhubarb	• Whole milk • Mozzarella (made with whole milk) • Full fat cheese (ex. sharp cheddar, swiss)

TRACKING APP

Carb counting is very important when learning keto. Cronometer App wins as the best place to learn and track your food. Other apps allow users to submit nutrition info without verification. More than once, I've depended upon the report from an app with false information.

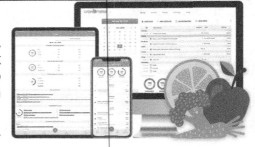

Inaccurate nutritional information can distract your progress. Cronometer verifies the nutrition data before allowing it into their database. Actual human beings check for accuracy first. Their staff is amazing.

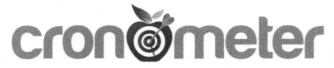

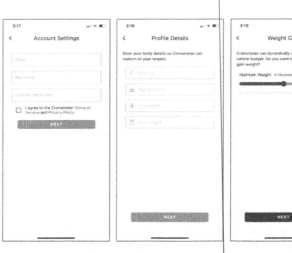

Step 1:

Download the free Cronometer App.

Step 2:

Set up account

Enter profile details as prompted.

I recommend adjusting these settings using a laptop or tablet.

Step 3:

UNDER SETTINGS, set your TARGETS to total carbs

Choose the KETO CALCULATOR (not fixed values or Macro Ratios). Select the Keto Calculator to the rigorous program. This will plot your protein to be 1.0 gram of protein for every kilogram of lean body mass. It will also keep your TOTAL carbohydrates at 20 grams per day.

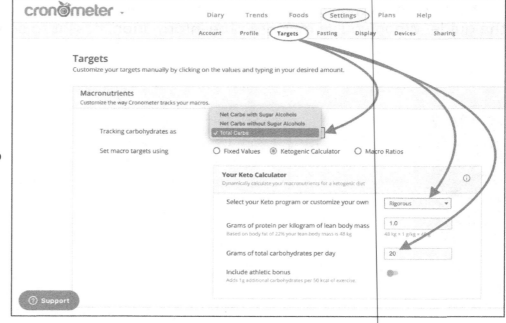

Step 4:

TRACK CARBS, NOT CALORIES

Under SETTINGS, select DISPLAY.

Slide the Calories Summary in Diary to OFF.

Summary column in Diary should be Carbs (Total)

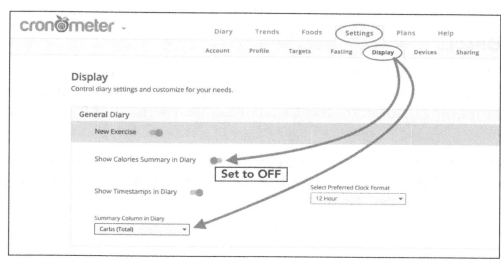

Step 5:

Scroll down on the display page to find nutrients.

The nutrition metrics will matter more in a month. You may want to track your intake of copper, iron, or Vitamin C.

Cronometer keeps a record of these tiny elements for any food entered.

Why is this important?

When you're eating keto, your food choices shift. For now, simply take notice of this feature. You will care more about this in the weeks ahead.

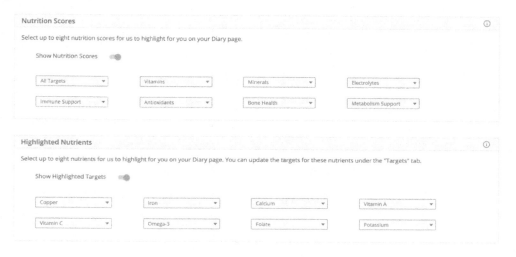

Track your carbs for three days before you start limiting them to 20 total carbs per day. If this is your second time around, track carbs for three days before starting AGAIN. Build your record of food using this app.

OTHER COOL FEATURES OF CRONOMETER APP:

ORACLE

The Oracle helps find foods tailored to your situation. Instruct it to find certain nutrients or suggest general food ideas that fit into your keto settings. When my patients advance to higher levels of keto, the Oracle teaches them what foods belong in their diet.

Nutrient Search: Here's an example of Oracle's foods with high magnesium.
Under FOODS, select Ask the Oracle. Set the nutrient to Magnesium, and rank the foods by "The Oracle." Because of the settings from the previous instructions, Oracle suggests only magnesium-rich keto options.

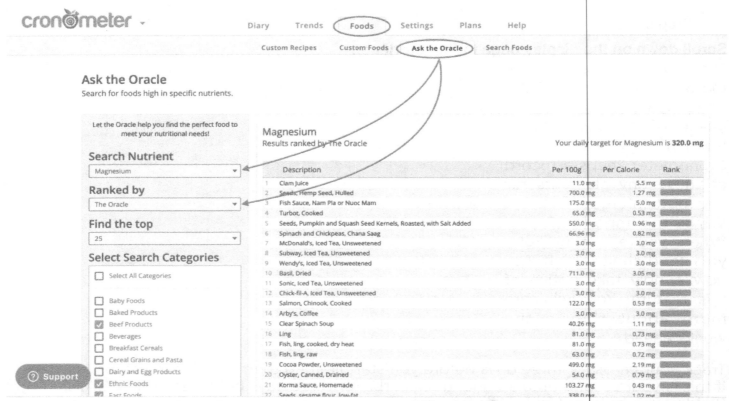

Oracle also curates a list of common foods for the items that best satisfy the constraints of your remaining targets for the day.

Select categories of food that please your palate. Oracle will do the rest. If you want to avoid eggs, tell Oracle.

Click a thumbs up to indicate the food you like. Teach oracle not to suggest certain foods by selecting a thumbs down.

ketoCONTINUUM **Workbook**

RED BEAKER MEANS BETTER DATA:

When adding food, search for the item generically— dropping brand names. High-Quality results are indicated with the red lab beaker icon.

The screenshot offers the example of Brazil nuts. Notice the highlight. A high-quality item identifies 76 listed nutrients found in Brazil nuts.[Look at the bottom of the screenshot.] Compare that with the branded version of Brazil nuts. Only 15 listed nutrients will be entered into your databank if you select the branded version of Brazil nuts.

Chose the one with the red beaker for better data.

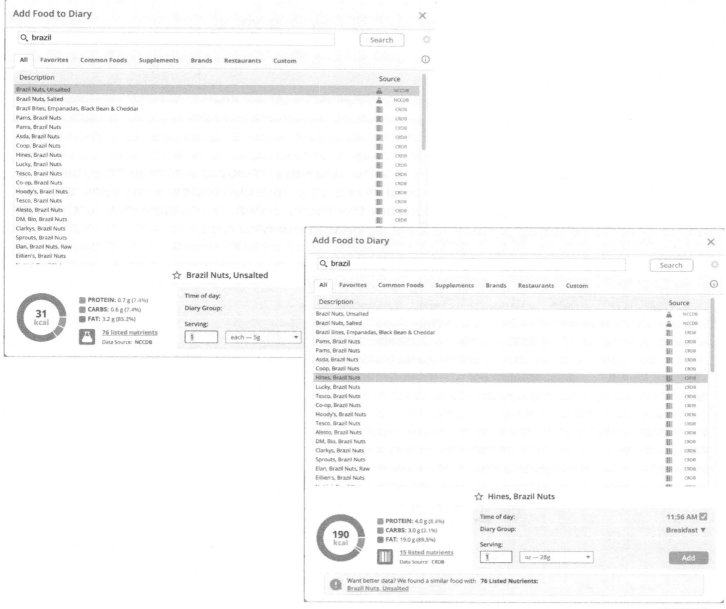

BARCODE SCANNER-

If items don't have a high-quality (red beaker) entry but have a barcode, scan the barcode. The item will show up immediately if it's in the databank. Rarely, an item is missing. If that occurs, take a picture of the nutrition label. Cronometer App will read the label and import all the nutrition information. No manual entries needed. This is a big time saver.

FASTING TIMER

Use the timer within the app to keep track of how long you've fasted.

COPY SELECTED ITEMS

An easy way to reduce the effort to log food is to copy and paste between days in the diary. This is especially helpful if you eat the same items day to day.

These screenshots show what it looks like to highlight multiple items in the diary then paste them in another day. While holding down the shift-button, click on each item you want. Then right-click and select copy from the menu. Move to the new day in the diary. Right-click and select paste. The items will appear in the new spot.

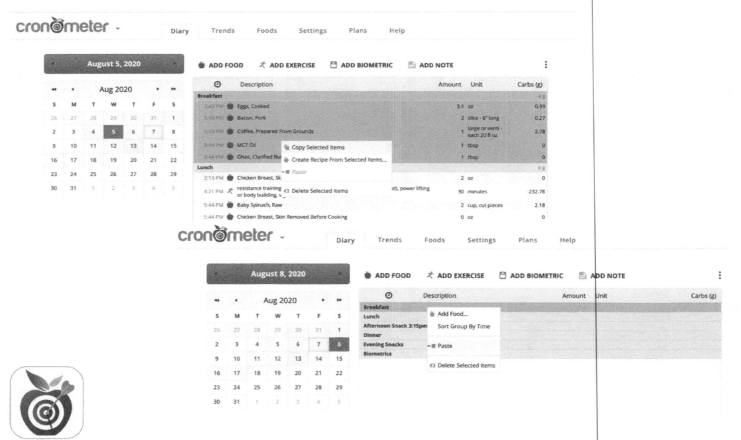

ketoCONTINUUM **Workbook**

COPY/PASTE ALL FOOD FROM CURRENT OR PREVIOUS DAY:

Use the "Copy Current Day" or "Copy Previous Day" options to duplicate the entire day's contents. Select "Copy Previous Day" to put everything from the day before into the current day. Or "Copy Current Day" to any day using the calendar and paste the contents there.

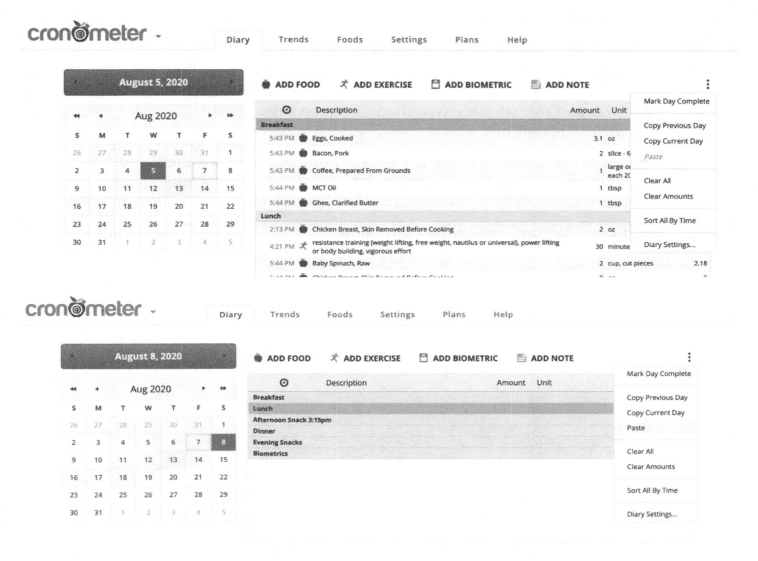

MEASURE WHAT MATTERS

This final section of 1.3 focuses on measurements. The first measurements can be done without a physician. The final chart offers several of the labs I follow in patients.

MEASUREMENTS WITHOUT A DOCTOR.

Take these measurements before you start.

1. **CARBS CONSUMED IN 24 HOURS**: Count your carbs before you start.

    a. For 3 days before starting, using your Cronometer App to keep track of your carbs. Do this BEFORE you start. If you are restarting the keto diet, do this BEFORE you restart. This will shed so much insight into your next two weeks. You will not regret this advice.

    b. Add them up before you start. Please do not skip this. It's profoundly important in predicting how well your continuum will go. If you eat more than 200 carbs per day, you are in the 200 Club. [See section 2.5 for 200 Club Instructions.]

Date	Food Diary before you change anything	Total Carbs
	Day 1	
	Day2	
	Day 3	

BMI CHART

WEIGHT

HEIGHT	120	130	140	150	160	170	180	190	200	210	220	230	240	250	260	270	280	290	300	310	320	330	340	360	380	400
5'0"	23	25	27	29	31	33	35	37	39	41	43	45	47	49	51	53	55	57	59	61	63	65	66	70	74	78
5'1"	23	25	27	28	30	32	34	36	38	40	42	44	45	47	49	51	53	55	57	59	61	62	64	68	71	75
5'2"	22	24	26	27	29	31	33	35	37	38	40	42	44	46	48	49	51	53	55	57	59	60	62	65	69	73
5'3"	21	23	25	27	28	30	32	34	36	37	39	41	43	44	46	48	50	51	53	55	57	59	60	63	67	70
5'4"	21	22	24	26	28	29	31	33	34	36	38	40	41	43	45	46	48	50	52	53	55	57	58	61	65	68
5'5"	20	22	23	25	27	28	30	32	33	35	37	38	40	42	43	45	47	48	50	52	53	55	56	60	63	67
5'6"	19	21	23	24	26	27	29	31	32	34	36	37	39	40	42	44	45	47	48	50	52	53	55	58	61	64
5'7"	19	20	22	24	25	27	28	30	31	33	34	36	38	39	41	42	44	46	47	49	50	52	53	56	60	63
5'8"	18	20	21	23	24	26	27	29	30	32	33	35	36	38	40	41	43	44	46	47	49	50	52	55	58	61
5'9"	18	19	21	22	24	25	27	28	30	31	32	34	35	37	38	40	41	43	44	46	47	49	50	53	56	59
5'10"	17	19	20	22	23	24	26	27	29	30	32	33	34	36	37	39	40	42	43	45	46	47	49	52	55	57
5'11"	17	18	20	21	22	24	25	27	28	29	31	32	33	35	36	38	39	41	42	43	45	46	47	50	53	56
6'0"	16	18	19	20	22	23	24	26	27	29	30	31	33	34	35	37	38	39	41	42	43	45	46	49	52	54
6'1"	16	17	19	20	21	22	24	25	26	28	29	30	32	33	34	36	37	38	40	41	42	44	45	48	50	53
6'2"	15	17	18	19	21	22	23	24	26	27	28	30	31	32	33	35	36	37	39	40	41	42	44	46	49	51
6'3"	15	16	18	19	20	21	22	24	25	26	28	29	30	31	33	34	35	36	38	39	40	41	43	45	48	50
6'4"	15	16	17	18	20	21	22	23	24	26	27	28	29	30	32	33	34	35	37	38	39	40	41	44	46	49
6'5"	14	16	17	18	19	20	21	23	24	25	26	27	29	30	31	32	33	34	36	37	38	39	40	43	45	47
6'6"	14	15	16	17	19	20	21	22	23	24	25	27	28	29	30	31	32	34	35	36	37	38	39	42	44	46
6'7"	14	15	16	17	18	19	20	21	23	24	25	26	27	28	29	30	32	33	34	35	36	37	38	41	43	45
6'8"	13	15	16	17	18	19	20	21	22	23	24	25	26	27	29	30	31	32	33	34	35	36	37	39	42	44
6'9"	13	14	15	16	17	18	19	20	21	23	24	25	26	27	28	29	30	31	32	33	34	35	36	39	41	43
6'10"	13	14	15	16	17	18	19	20	21	22	23	24	25	26	27	28	29	30	31	32	34	35	35	38	40	42

HEIGHT

Underweight:
BMI = less than 18.5

Normal weight:
BMI = 18.5 to 24.9

Overweight:
BMI = 25 to 29.9

Obesity Class I:
BMI = 30 to 34.9

Obesity Class II:
BMI = 35 to 39.9

Extreme Obesity
BMI = 40 and above

The following worksheet is very valuable. Of course, it's only valuable if you fill it out. I encourage patients to record these measurements every 6 months. You can do it more often, but the improvement process takes time. Skin tags, neck circumference, and fasting glucose take time to improve.

2. Fill in the Worksheet

a. <u>Date</u>: Don't skip this. Document the date when you measure these. (Even if you started the diet already ... Do this!)

b. <u>Blood Pressure</u>: Be sure to relax the muscles of your arm and have the cuff at the same level as your heart.

c. <u>BMI (Body Mass Index)</u>: Find your WEIGHT AND HEIGHT on the BMI chart on the previous page. Enter the correlating BMI into its column on the worksheet.

d. <u>Morning Fasting Blood Sugar</u>: Be sure to check it FIRST THING in the morning. As soon as you are done with the bathroom, prick your finger and check your blood glucose.

e. <u>Waistline</u>: Men's Goal: <40 in   Women's Goal: <35 in

f. <u>Neck Circumference</u>: A neck circumference greater than 17 inches predicts sleep apnea. Measure it.

g. <u>Shin Thumbprint</u>: Push your thumb into your shin and hold for 30 seconds. Lift your hand and see if there is a print left behind.

    0= No indentation in your shin.
    1= A mild indentation.
    2= Between mild and severe impression.
    3= A severe indentation.

h. <u>Skin Tags</u>: Check your armpits, the skin around your neck, and in other folds such as your groin. Add up the total number of skin tags you have. These are caused by years of high insulin. Keto-chemistry reverses this problem.

MEASUREMENT CHART

Date	Blood Pressure	BMI	Morning Fasting Glucose	Waistline	Neck Circumference	Thumb Shin-Print	Skin Tags
	<130/85	<25	<100	<40 in <35 in	<17 in	None	0

MEASUREMENTS FROM THE MEDICAL TEAM

1. HGA1C: Also called hbA1C-

Measures the average of the blood sugars over the past 3 months. Check your old lab reports to see if this has been done. Alternatively, you can order a home kit from your local pharmacy or off Amazon. https://amzn.to/37eg0b5 . The kits cost about $150 and allow you to test yourself 10 times. The process has limitations such as storing the kit in the refrigerator and carefully following the multi-step process. Also, replacement strips are not available -- an entirely new kit and strips need to be purchased after the 10 tests are used. The results are rather accurate. This test offers great insight into the state of your sugars over the past months.

HbA1c TEST SCORE

HbA1c	mg/dL PRECEDING 3-MONTH AVERAGE BLOOD GLUCOSE	mmol/L PRECEDING 3-MONTH AVERAGE BLOOD GLUCOSE	
4.0	68	3.8	REVERSING AGING
4.5	82	4.5	
5.0	97	5.4	
5.5	111	6.1	
6.0	126	7	FASTER AGING
6.5	140	7.8	
7.0	154	8.6	
7.5	169	9.4	DANGER
8.0	183	10.1	
8.5	197	10.9	
9.0	212	11.8	
9.5	226	12.5	
10.0	240	13.3	
10.5	255	14.1	
11.0	269	14.9	
11.5	283	15.7	
12.0	298	16.5	
12.5	312	18.1	
13.0	326	14.5	
13.5	340	18.9	

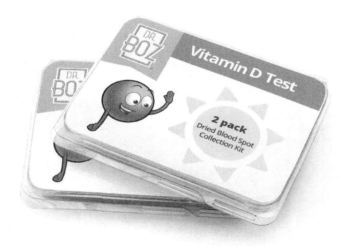

2. Vitamin D Test: http://on.bozmd.com/vitD

25-hydroxy Vitamin D is the actual name of the lab test. Check old lab reports to see if you've had it measured in the past. I instruct my patients to measure it themselves. In fact, I ask them to measure it before starting and repeat after 4 months of keto.

The HOME Vitamin D tests are easy to do and cost about $50 for each measurement. In comparison, the cost of the Vitamin D test at the clinic laboratory ranges from $75-$200. The home test involves pricking your finger and filling up the circle on a special spongy card with drips of your blood. This dried blot of blood is mailed to the processing lab and accurately reports your Vitamin D level. The home testing empowers the patient to take ownership of their care.

3. Omega 3 Index Complete Test

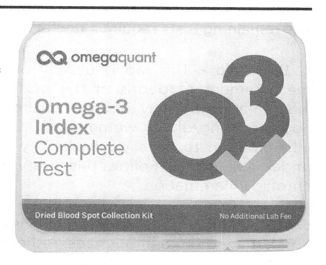

http://on.bozmd.com/Omega3
This test costs about $100 and reports the types of fat found within the lining of your red blood cells including the Omega 3 Index and the Trans Fat Index.

Omega 3 Index:

An Omega-3 Index in the range of 8-12% is one indicator of better overall health. These ranges were derived from thousands of individuals whose RBC samples were analyzed for the Omega-3 Index.

Like the Vitamin D home test, a kit to prick your finger accompanies a special sponge card. Once your blood has been absorbed into the card, you are instructed to mail it back to the lab. The type of fats found in the "skin" of your red blood cells is measured and reported back. The best fat is Omega 3 and is reported to you as the Omega3 Index.

An Omega-3 Index above 8% helps maintain heart, brain, eye, and joint health. The best way to increase your Omega-3 Index is to eat more omega-3 fatty acids, specifically EPA and DHA. These are found primarily in fish, especially "oily" fish such as sardines, mackerel, and salmon. They can also be obtained from dietary supplements (fish, krill, cod liver, and algal oils).

Trans Fat Index:

Omega 3 fats reign as the healthiest fats to eat; trans fats are the worst. The Trans Fat Index is the amount of industrially produced trans fats that are in your red blood cell membranes. These levels of trans fats reflect levels in the diet — the more you eat, the higher the trans fats are in the blood. Historically, Americans ate too much trans fat, but over the last several years the food industry has steadily removed trans fats from many products. In fact, since 2009, the average Trans Fat Index should be less than <1%.

The remaining tests require a doctor's order.

4. Uric Acid - This lab is usually ordered to assess gout in patients. Think of it as a measurement of debris in the body. Similarly, I teach patients to judge their chronic inflammation by way of their serum uric acid. Measurements of serum uric acid levels above 6.0 mg/dL for women and 7.0 mg/dL for men warn of enough debris and chronic inflammation to have gout. Healthy bodies have uric acid under 5.0 mg/dL, preferably under 4.5 mg/dL. Follow this every 6 - 12 months to see how well you have reversed chronic inflammation.

5. ALT - Alanine transaminase (ALT) is an enzyme found mostly in the liver. When liver cells are damaged the number rises. Although there are many causes of elevated liver enzymes, I follow this as a means to measure fatty liver. When this number is greater than 25, you likely have excess fat in your liver cells. Follow this number to assess if you have "emptied" excess fat from your liver.

6. hsCRP — (See Chapter 22 for interpretations)

7. CAC - (See Chapter 22 for interpretations) I recommend ONE screening test of Coronary Artery Calcium (CAC) for my patients who have never taken a statin to reduce cholesterol. If you've taken a statin for a year, this test will always come back elevated. Save your money. I am not a huge fan of following this test over time. If patients really want to know their heart risk, I encourage the Omega-3 Index.

8. Ferritin - Ferritin reflects iron in the body. I like to see the ferritin greater than 50 ng/mL when we are trying to repair a body — especially a brain.

9. Triglycerides/HDL - Divide your triglycerides by your HDL number found on a screening cholesterol panel. This number should be less than 1.5. This is the most useful part of the cholesterol screening panel. Focus on this ratio.

Do not plan to repeat these tests until you have steadily produced keto-chemistry for at least 12 weeks. Let me clarify: Spend 12 weeks with proven ketosis. Then consider re-measuring some of these labs. Not before that.

LABORATORY CHART

Date	HgA1c	Omega 3 Index	Trans Fat Index	Vit D-25 Hydroxy	ALT	hsCRP	Uric Acid	CAC	Ferritin	TG/HDL mg/dl (mmol/L)
	<5.0 %	>8%	<1%	>50 ng/mL	<40u/L	<1.0 mg/L	<5.0 mg/ dL	<100	>50 ng/mL	<1.5 (<0.65)

1.4 Cupboard Therapy

THROW AWAY THE PINE NEEDLES:

Clean out your cupboards. Clean out the pine needle-type fuel.
Don't start grocery shopping. Start with throwing away. Do not stop tossing items until the shelves in the fridge and pantry shine with empty spaces.

When patients join my local support group, I encourage them to complete this within two days.

I OFFER TWO OPTIONS:

1. Send me a picture of your cupboards and fridge.

    OR

2. I will visit your home and look at the cupboards by the end of the week.

Accountability. The cupboard-check helps you take action.

Be accountable for the change you want. Start with removing temptations.

The first two weeks of a ketogenic diet can feel like withdrawal. Do not underestimate the power of craving for carbohydrates. Before you begin, empty the cupboards.
Remove fattening foods.

Clean up the environment when you're feeling, "normal." It may take two to three weeks before you use up all your pine-needles and get through the withdrawal from carbs. Ask a friend to come over to your house and help you—one of those people on your list from the last chapter.

How do you know which food items to throw away?

Start with the label.

Look at the carbs per serving. You get 20 total carbs per day. So any item with a high level of carbohydrates or sugars needs to go. Period.
Highly processed food hits the trash. Throw it. My kids helped. I taught them to count the number of ingredients in the product. If there were more than eight ingredients in the product, we called that, "Highly processed food." After that, we tossed everything made with flour, rice, corn, or sugar.
Opened items went to the burning barrel. Unopened items filled the box for the community food pantry.

Removing temptations from our home was therapeutic for the entire family.

FATTENING FOODS:

THE FOLLOWING FOODS ARE ALL HIGH IN CARBOHYDRATES AND SHOULD BE REMOVED FROM YOUR SIGHT.

Bread: Anything made from wheat flour, white flour, pumpernickel flour, rye flour, tortillas, waffles, rolls, pasta, raisin bread. Use finely ground almonds (almond flour) or coconuts (coconut flour) as a substitution. Be careful with these substitution flours. They stimulate insulin more than you'd think.

Cereals and Grains: bran cereals, cooked cereals, stuffing, unsweetened cereals, cornmeal, couscous, granola, grape-nuts, grits, pasta, quinoa, rice, brown rice, shredded wheat, sugar cereals.

Fruit Juices: All juices associated with fruit, except lemon or lime juice in small quantities.

Fruit: apple, applesauce, dried apples, apricots, bananas, cantaloupe, cherries, grapefruit, grapes, kiwi, honeydew, mangoes, mandarin oranges, nectarines, oranges, papaya, peaches, pears, pineapples, raisins, tangerines, dried fruit.

Beans, Peas, and Nuts: baked beans, black beans, peas, garbanzo beans, pinto beans, kidney beans, white beans, split beans, black-eyed beans, Lima beans, cashew nuts, chestnuts, tofu, soybeans.

Milk: nonfat milk, chocolate milk, evaporated milk, skim milk, whole milk, soy milk, nonfat yogurt.

Carb-Filled-Vegetables: corn, peas, potatoes, squash, yams, sweet potatoes.

Snacks: animal crackers, goldfish crackers, graham crackers, oyster crackers, popped popcorn, pretzels, sandwich crackers, chips, tortilla chips, potato chips, french fries.

Sweets: Anything with sugar, honey, or other sweeteners. Cake, biscuits, brownies, candy, chocolate, cookies, sauces, donuts, ice cream, jams, jellies, ketchup, pie, frosting.

Take a picture of clean cupboards. POST IT TO THE GROUP!

☐ DONE _____ (date)

1.5 TROUBLE CLUBS

DR. CLUB

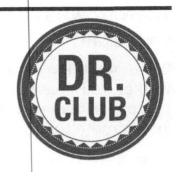

Who should see a doctor before starting ketogenic nutrition?
See a physician before you start:

#1 If you take blood pressure medications

#2 If you have less than 25% of your kidney function

#3 If you take Coumadin (warfarin)

#4 If you take a diuretic prescription— commonly known as a pee pill

#5 If you inject insulin daily

#6 If you drink alcohol daily, beware.

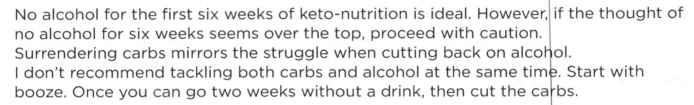

No alcohol for the first six weeks of keto-nutrition is ideal. However, if the thought of no alcohol for six weeks seems over the top, proceed with caution.
Surrendering carbs mirrors the struggle when cutting back on alcohol.
I don't recommend tackling both carbs and alcohol at the same time. Start with booze. Once you can go two weeks without a drink, then cut the carbs.

If you said YES to any of the above problems, you are in the Dr. Club.

200 CLUB

Track your carbs using the Cronometer App for three days before starting.
Do you eat more than 200 total carbs per day?
    If you do, you are in the 200 Club.

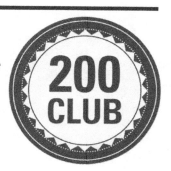

200 CLUB + DR. CLUB

LET'S START AGAIN

If you are in the 200 Club or the Dr. Club...Stop. Slow down.

You need closer observation than just reading a book or watching a video.

Skip to the plan outlined in the "LET'S START AGAIN" paragraph in section 2.5.

ketoCONTINUUM

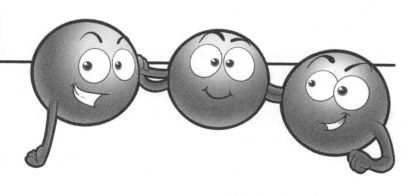

SECTION

2

KETO FIRST WEEK

2.1.   Day 1: Begin

2.2.   Day 2: Eat Fat

2.3.   Day 3: Pray for Pink

2.4.   Day 4: Oh Poop!

2.5.   No Ketones: End of Day 4

2.6.   How to Spend Time During Setback or Stall

2.7.   Day 5: Magnesium

2.8.   Day 6: Calories & Cravings

2.9.   Meetings & Mirror Neurons

BozMD.com

2.1. DAY 1: BEGIN

What time did you eat yesterday?
Add that time to the box.

:

The first 48 hours are the most difficult. Set a timer for 48 hours.
Follow these 3 steps.

STEP 1: NO SUGAR. NO STARCH. HIGH FAT.
Say those words out loud.

Again. No sugar. No starch. High fat.

BREAKFAST IDEAS:
- Eggs & bacon. If you scramble the eggs, add FULL-fat cheese, not low-fat cheese.
- A bowl of ground hamburger soaked in butter. Eat until you are full.

Do not go grocery shopping yet. If your house has no eggs, ground hamburger, or bacon, grab a drive-through breakfast.
Order two sausage patties with NO bun. Ask for egg and cheese in the middle.
You read that right. In the drive-through order, "Sausage and egg breakfast sandwich. Hold the bun. Use two sausage patties as the bun with egg and cheese in the middle."
Ask them to wrap it like a breakfast sandwich. This is cheap, easy, and TOTALLY KETO.

STEP 2: TWENTY. 20.

20 TOTAL GRAMS OF CARBOHYDRATES PER DAY.

The only thing I want you to count is carbohydrates. Not calories. Not grams of fiber, fat, or protein. Use the Cronometer app for the best results. Use the chart on the following page to keep track.

STEP 3: PEE ON A KETONE-STICK

WHAT MAY I DRINK = NOTHING SWEET

The first few weeks require a high supply of fat in the absence of carbs. One easy way to add fat is to drink it. Popular keto-coffee drinks add heavy cream, butter, coconut oil, or MCT C8:C10 oil into the coffee. Your taste buds will enjoy it. The first phase of keto depends upon adequate fat.

Pour on the fat! Do. Not. Skip. The. Fat.

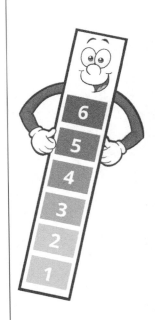

CHART YOUR CARBS:

TIME	FOOD	TOTAL CARBS	HOW DO YOU FEEL?
8:00 am	Hard Boiled Eggs 6	26	Full

TOTAL CARBS =

2.2 Day 2: Eat Fat

When you wake up, head to the bathroom where you placed those Ketone (PeeTone) strips. Pee on a strip. Is it pink? Register the time and your PeeTone strip color on the chart each time you test today.

Pink PeeTone Strip means KETONES.

You made ketones! In fact, you made a few extra. That's okay. Your kidney flushed the extra ketones into your urine and you voided it out. Pink PeeTone strips tell you that your bloodstream holds ketones now. Yesterday, it did not. This is progress.

White PeeTone Strip means NO KETONES.

If your strip does not turn pink, there are no ketones in your urine or your strips are bad. PeeTone strips go bad when exposed to the air too long. PeeTones come inside a dark, tightly sealed container to prevent them from degrading.

Eat fat for breakfast, lunch, and dinner.

We must awaken your cells that help absorb fat. Low-fat diets put them to sleep. Excess insulin makes them sluggish. Awaken them by eating fat without carbs. The oily slick inside your mouth will fade when your parotid gland improves the way it makes enzymes. Your gut will improve the way it absorbs fat too.

This is the toughest day. Expect cravings and the desire to stick to your routine eating habits. If you crave food 6 times today, eat 6 times. Keep eating until you are full, but ONLY eat fatty foods with nearly zero carbs. I want you as close to zero carbs as you can get for these first days. We MUST lower your insulin.

Food choices

Choose foods containing salt and fat. I'll list just a few of your many choices. Cheese + pepperoni + avocado + meat sticks + pork rinds + pink salt crystals.

Dip the foods in mayonnaise/mustard sauce. Dip them in sour cream with hot sauce or sour cream mixed with ranch dressing powder.

HAVE YOU PEED YOUR FIRST KETONE?

☐ YES! Time: _____ How long did it take? _____ ☐ NO

STRUGGLES ON DAY 2

DRINK OPTIONS

Coffee with heavy whipping cream—sprinkle in a little salt. That may sound gross to some. It took me over four years to figure out the importance of salt. Learn from me.

Salt matters. Salt is critical to helping you through these first days. It will remain a vital part of this lifestyle. Any way you sneak a little salt into the plan is a WIN. I prefer Redmonds Salt.

Add water—always a great option. Salted water is even better.

Pique Tea—a brand of instant tea that does not taste like instant tea. I like fresh brewed iced tea, NOT instant. Pique Tea is the only exception I have found. I truly love the taste of their freeze-dried, powdered tea.

No protein shakes. No smoothies filled with green. We must correct your chemistry. Those things mess it up.

See the Rx for Beta-Hydroxybutyrate in Section 2.5 for best practices regarding ketones-in-a-can. This transition can be rough for some. folks. Exogenous ketones will help the transition.

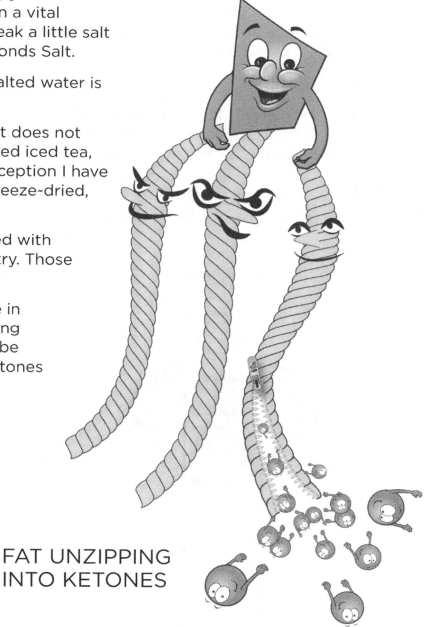

FAT UNZIPPING
INTO KETONES

CHECK YOUR BLOOD PRESSURE

Blood pressure fluctuates on the first two weeks of a ketogenic diet. Keep an eye on how it changes. Several days of blood pressure trending up or down will settle into a pattern at about 7-10 days. Keep the chart to show your doctor what happened.

TAKE AN EPSOM SALT BATH

See Section 1.1. Reread your your Why.
Take time to reflect on your struggle. Be gentle to yourself. It's catchy. When you treat yourself kindly, it spreads to others.

BOWEL MOVEMENTS

A change in your bowel habits is expected when starting ketogenic nutrition. Did your bowels move today? Document that in the chart. If they did not move, swallow a cap full of the milk of magnesia. Keep track of your bowel movements for the first several days.

GO TO BED

Congratulations, you made it through day two!

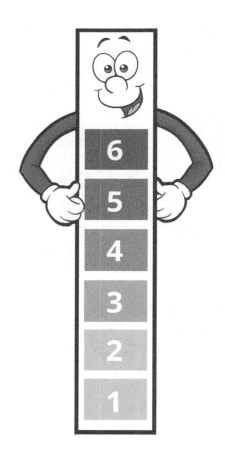

It's not uncommon to repeat Day 2. Date the first time you do Day 2. Hopefully you will not fall off the wagon, but if you do, date the second time around too.
Count your "TOTAL CARBS" and document the time along the second column.

DAY 2 DATE	TIME	BLOOD PRESSURE	HEART RATE	PEETONE STRIP COLOR	TOTAL CARBS	BOWEL ACTIVITY
				0 1 2 3 4 5 6		
				0 1 2 3 4 5 6		
				0 1 2 3 4 5 6		
				0 1 2 3 4 5 6		
				0 1 2 3 4 5 6		
				0 1 2 3 4 5 6		
				0 1 2 3 4 5 6		
				0 1 2 3 4 5 6		
				0 1 2 3 4 5 6		
				0 1 2 3 4 5 6		
				0 1 2 3 4 5 6		
				0 1 2 3 4 5 6		
				0 1 2 3 4 5 6		
				0 1 2 3 4 5 6		
				0 1 2 3 4 5 6		
				0 1 2 3 4 5 6		
				0 1 2 3 4 5 6		
				1 2 3 4 5 6		
				3 4 5 6		
				3 4 5 6		

2.3 DAY 3: PRAY FOR PINK

MORNING RITUAL

MAKE THIS YOUR MORNING RITUAL:

1. Check your ketone urine strip when you wake up and go to the bathroom.

2. Put 3-4 more strips in your pocket.

3. Each time you pee, check your PeeTones.

4. Salt all food for today and tomorrow.

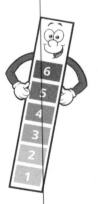

Have you peed your first ketone?

☐ YES! Time: _____   How long did it take? _____   ☐ NO

DAY 3 CHART

DAY 3 DATE	TIME	BLOOD PRESSURE	HEART RATE	PEETONE STRIP COLOR	TOTAL CARBS	BOWEL ACTIVITY
				0 1 2 3 4 5 6		
				0 1 2 3 4 5 6		
				0 1 2 3 4 5 6		
				0 1 2 3 4 5 6		
				0 1 2 3 4 5 6		
				0 1 2 3 4 5 6		
				0 1 2 3 4 5 6		
				0 1 2 3 4 5 6		
				0 1 2 3 4 5 6		
				0 1 2 3 4 5 6		
				0 1 2 3 4 5 6		
				0 1 2 3 4 5 6		
				0 1 2 3 4 5 6		
				0 1 2 3 4 5 6		
				0 1 2 3 4 5 6		
				0 1 2 3 4 5 6		
				0 1 2 3 4 5 6		
				0 1 2 3 4 5 6		
				0 1 2 3 4 5 6		
				0 1 2 3 4 5 6		

2.4 DAY 4: OH POOP!

Fill out this chart on your forth day.

DAY 4 DATE	TIME	BLOOD PRESSURE	HEART RATE	PEETONE STRIP COLOR	TOTAL CARBS	BOWEL ACTIVITY
				0 1 2 3 4 5 6		
				0 1 2 3 4 5 6		
				0 1 2 3 4 5 6		
				0 1 2 3 4 5 6		
				0 1 2 3 4 5 6		
				0 1 2 3 4 5 6		
				0 1 2 3 4 5 6		
				0 1 2 3 4 5 6		
				0 1 2 3 4 5 6		
				0 1 2 3 4 5 6		
				0 1 2 3 4 5 6		
				0 1 2 3 4 5 6		
				0 1 2 3 4 5 6		
				0 1 2 3 4 5 6		
				0 1 2 3 4 5 6		
				0 1 2 3 4 5 6		
				0 1 2 3 4 5 6		
				0 1 2 3 4 5 6		
				0 1 2 3 4 5 6		

BOWELS: TOO SLOW [CONSTIPATION]

Ketosis-induced constipation is an expected complication. Due to the decreased volume of food, your bowels slow down. Additionally, the water flushed out of your body the first-week results in harder, slow-moving stools.

1. DRINK SALTY WATER. ALSO CALLED SOLÉ WATER

Recipe for Solé Water: Add two large sea salt crystals (about the size of a lime) fill with water. As the crystals dissolve over the next several days, use the salted water for cooking, adding to drinks like tea or coffee.

2. CHIA SEEDS TO THE RESCUE. (SEE BELOW)

3. MILK OF MAGNESIA

This cheap, accessible liquid adds magnesium to your body & helps flush your bowels along. Don't be afraid to use this the first couple of weeks in conjunction with Chia seeds.

4. ABDOMINAL MASSAGE

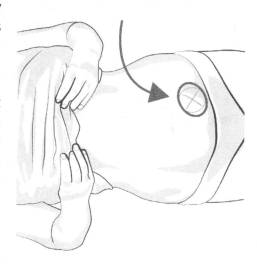

Every nursing student knows what this is: massage the left lower quadrant of the abdomen when the patient is constipated. I teach my patients how to do this to themselves. Constipation feels awful. Learning to stimulate the movement of your bowels by massaging the abdomen can save you from aches and pains. While laying on your back, bend your knees to decrease the tension on your abdomen. Press both hands (one on top of the other) into the area between your left leg and your belly button. [See drawing. Aim for the circle.]

Slowly press down, massaging back and forth. When I demonstrate this to patients, I place their fingertips in the area of the circle first and then my hands on top of theirs. We start by rocking the fingertips into the abdomen. The added pressure using both hands compresses the abdomen by a couple of inches.

Push hard enough to stimulate the bowel muscles to contract. Massage for 3-5 minutes. This will help with constipation.

5. EXOGENOUS KETONES (BHB)

Yes - Ketones-In-A-Can have another benefit. Ketones-In-A-Can are salts. Swallow a bunch of ketone salts at once and you flush out your backside. Some ketones will get absorbed into your circulation. Those absorbed ketones will help you but expect loose stools if you drink exogenous ketones too quickly.

6. ADD THE CABBAGE

Cabbage can be a great way to transition from Hi-carb to low carb. Initially, slice cabbage and eat raw with dressing added to the greens. Several days later smother with butter and broil in the oven. The best longterm keto-cabbage is the fermented style: sauerkraut.

7. CHIA SEEDS FOR SLOW BOWELS

When you ate high-carbs or high-fiber food, your bowel depended upon the bulk of food to stretch your colon. Once it stretched enough, you triggered the bowel muscles to contract. Squeezing against the bulk or volume trained your bowel to depend upon the stretch of your colon to trigger those muscles. Removing those carb-filled, hight-fiber foods removed the stretch factor your bowels depended upon. Chia seeds and saltwater can expand inside the colon and be used to stretch the diameter of the colon without high carbs. Use the chart below to add the right amount of seeds to trigger your bowel.

Use each square in the chart below to mark the hours and doses of Chia seeds. Place an X in each square as you follow this protocol. Find the dose of chia seeds needed to stretch your bowel.

	CHIA SEEDS FOR BOWELS TOO SLOW: TAPE ON											
Date	1 Tbsp	1 Tbsp	1 Tbsp	1 Tbsp	1 Tbsp	1 Tbsp	1 Tbsp	1 Tbsp	1 Tbsp	1 Tbsp	1 Tbsp	1 Tbsp
	Dose 1	Dose 2	Dose 3	Dose 4	Dose 5	Dose 6	Dose 7	Dose 8	Dose 9	Dose 10	Dose 11	Dose 12
Time												
	Dose 13	Dose 14	Dose 15	Dose 16	Dose 17	Dose 18	Dose 19	Dose 20	Dose 21	Dose 22	Dose 23	Dose 24
Time												

- Swallow one tablespoon of dry chia seeds every hour with several ounces of salty water. Document the time of each spoonful.
  - o Place the seeds in your mouth.
  - o Chew a couple of times and wash them down with a glass of salty water.
  - o Be sure the water has salt. I prefer Solé Water.
- Add another tablespoon every hour while awake.
- Keep going until you have a bowel movement.
- Tally the number of tablespoons you swallowed before your bowels moved.
- The total number sets your daily chia-seed dose for the next day.
  - o For example, if you had 12 tablespoons before your bowels responded, take 12 tablespoons the next day.

- o Instead of dosing seeds hourly, take 1/2 the dose first thing in the morning and the other half at noon.
- After three days at the dose, decrease by one tablespoon. Continue dropping one tablespoon every few days.

THIS PROTOCOL WORKS BECAUSE:

The Chia-Seed Protocol works to retrain your bowels to contract without the "trick" of stretching them. Squeezing against the bulk of fiber made your bowel dependent upon the stretch of the colon to trigger the muscles to move the stools.

Healthy, uninflamed colons don't require this stretch stimulus to move the stools. Heathy bowels are coated with a thick layer of slime. A small contraction easily slides the stools.

- Fiber stretches the colon. So do chia seeds.
- Dry chia seeds don't raise your blood sugar.
- The gentle decline of seeds while replacing water and salt makes for a great remedy.

Life without fiber is possible. Stick with keto chemistry and your poop problems will resolve.

DON'T COUNT THE CARBS IN CHIA SEEDS WHEN USING THE PROTOCOL.

Here are three reasons why:

1. The seeds end up flushed down the toilet.
2. They do not cause a significant insulin response.
3. The folks who need the seeds should use them without fear of overshooting the 20 total carbs. When bowel problems linger, students fall off the keto wagon. Use the chia seed protocol with the end in mind.

HERE IS AN EXTRA CHART IN CASE YOU NEED TO REPEAT THIS PROTOCOL:

CHIA SEEDS FOR BOWELS TOO SLOW: TAPE ON											
Date	1 Tbsp	1 Tbsp	1 Tbsp	1 Tbsp	1 Tbsp	1 Tbsp	1 Tbsp	1 Tbsp	1 Tbsp	1 Tbsp	1 Tbsp
	Dose 1	Dose 2	Dose 3	Dose 4	Dose 5	Dose 6	Dose 7	Dose 8	Dose 9	Dose 10	Dose 11	Dose 12
Time											
	Dose 13	Dose 14	Dose 15	Dose 16	Dose 17	Dose 18	Dose 19	Dose 20	Dose 21	Dose 22	Dose 23	Dose 24
Time											

Use this chart to taper your dose:

Day 1 = take your full chia-seed dose with salty water.

Day 2 = Subtract one tablespoon from yesterday's dose. Continue tapering by one tablespoon per day.

CHIA SEEDS TAPER OFF				
Day of Protocol	Morning Dose	Noon Dose	Bowel movement?	Notes
Day 1	7 Tbsp	7 Tbsp	Yes / No	
Day 2	7 Tbsp	6 Tbsp	Yes / No	
Day 3	6 Tbsp	6 Tbsp	Yes / No	
Day 4	6 Tbsp	5 Tbsp	Yes / No	
Day 5	5 Tbsp	5 Tbsp	Yes / No	
Day 6	5 Tbsp	4 Tbsp	Yes / No	
Day 7	4 Tbsp	4 Tbsp	Yes / No	
Day 8	4 Tbsp	3 Tbsp	Yes / No	
Day 9	3 Tbsp	3 Tbsp	Yes / No	
Day 10	3 Tbsp	2 Tbsp	Yes / No	
Day 11	2 Tbsp	2 Tbsp	Yes / No	
Day 12	2 Tbsp	1 Tbsp	Yes / No	
Day 13	2 Tbsp		Yes / No	
Day 14	1 Tbsp		Yes / No	

ketoCONTINUUM Workbook

Here is an extra chart in case you need to repeat this protocol:

CHIA SEEDS TAPER OFF				
Day of Protocol	**Morning Dose**	**Noon Dose**	**Bowel movement?**	**Notes**
Day 1	7 Tbsp	7 Tbsp	Yes / No	
Day 2	7 Tbsp	6 Tbsp	Yes / No	
Day 3	6 Tbsp	6 Tbsp	Yes / No	
Day 4	6 Tbsp	5 Tbsp	Yes / No	
Day 5	5 Tbsp	5 Tbsp	Yes / No	
Day 6	5 Tbsp	4 Tbsp	Yes / No	
Day 7	4 Tbsp	4 Tbsp	Yes / No	
Day 8	4 Tbsp	3 Tbsp	Yes / No	
Day 9	3 Tbsp	3 Tbsp	Yes / No	
Day 10	3 Tbsp	2 Tbsp	Yes / No	
Day 11	2 Tbsp	2 Tbsp	Yes / No	
Day 12	2 Tbsp	1 Tbsp	Yes / No	
Day 13	2 Tbsp		Yes / No	
Day 14	1 Tbsp		Yes / No	

BOWELS: TOO FAST [DIARRHEA]

Diarrhea following a meal of high fat is not normal. Often the flush of stool means your gut needs to heal. Diarrhea associated with a high fat diet means you are failing to absorb fat. Pooping the fat into the toilet has deadly consequences if left untreated. Talk to your doctor about this problem.

... and follow these tips:

1. **LICK THE SPOON**

    a. Add C8:C10 to the list of things to swallow. This unique fat requires no bile, no pancreatic enzymes, and no "digestion" to get into your circulation. If fats cause explosive diarrhea, your gut lining needs to heal. Lead the healing with this unique oil: C8:C10 MCT

        i. Begin with ONE soft-gel. Bite into the soft-gel and swallow the oil. If that causes distress, do not increase the dose until your gut has healed enough to use this oil.

        ii. Increase slowly to 10 soft-gels per day. This will help heal a gut that is damaged from chronic inflammation and bacterial overgrowth.

        iii. Once you can tolerate 10 soft-gels, consider adding the oil to your coffee or hot drink in the mornings.

2. **CHIA SEEDS**

    a. As with constipation, this protocol works from inside the tunnel of your intestines. The Chia Seeds absorb extra liquid in your stools and slow down the flush from your backside.

    b. Start the Chia Seed protocol. Unlike keto-induced-constipation, keto-diarrhea will not go away until the problem is fixed. If you taper off of chia seeds, and the diarrhea returns, see your doctor.

    c. Solé Water: Continue adding salt water when swallowing chia seeds.

3. **Fast:**

    There is no better antidote for a gut that is misbehaving than fasting. Stop all food for 36 hours. Sip on salty water. Preferably Redmond's Real salt.

4. **Consider a medical visit with a specialist for fat malabsorption.**

DIARRHEA CHIA SEED PROTOCOL:

After each loose bowel movement, swallow the associated dose of Chia seeds.

	CHIA SEEDS FOR BOWELS TOO FAST: TAPE ON									
Date	1 TBSP	2 TBSPs	3 TBSPs	4 TBSPs	5 TBSPs	6 TBSPs	7 TBSPs	8 TBSPs	9 TBSPs	10 TBSPs
	loose stool 1	loose stool 2	loose stool 3	loose stool 4	loose stool 5	loose stool 6	loose stool 7	loose stool 8	loose stool 9	loose stool 10
Total number TBSPs of chia seeds	1 total	3 total	6 total	10 total	15 total	21 total	28 total	36 total	45 total	55 total

If you get to the end of that row (10 tablespoons of chia seeds) and still have diarrhea, add Loperamide AND GO SEE A DOCTOR.

2.5 NO KETONES: END OF DAY 4

If you don't have pink PeeTone strips by day 4, something is wrong.

It might be:

1. **YOUR PEETONE STRIPS ARE BAD.**

   a. Double-check your PeeTone strips. Are they bad? Fresh air and time deactivate the sponge at the tip of the PeeTone strip. ANSWER: Get new strips.

2. **YOU'RE EATING MORE THAN 20 CARBOHYDRATES**

   a. Don't beat yourself up if you failed to keep the total carb number under 20. Life has seasons.

   b. ANSWER: Get the Cronometer App. Measure accurately with Cronometer for at least 3 days.

3. **YOU'RE DRINKING TOO MUCH ALCOHOL.**

   a. When alcohol is present, you stop burning ketones and glucose. Place all 3 fuel options (glucose, ketones, and alcohol) in front of hungry mitochondria and alcohol burns first, followed by ketones, and then carbs.

   b. ANSWER: Ideally, stop the alcohol before stopping carbs. Letting go of both chemicals at the same time proves difficult. Not impossible, but pretty tricky. Your brain and body chemistry needs time to reset after removing each of these chemicals. If it seems unlikely to say goodbye to booze, shift to no carb alcohol. Use distilled alcohol, not beer. Distilled booze drips out of a distillery from six fermenting options as Brandy, Gin, Rum, Tequila, Vodka, and Whiskey. Limit yourself to 3 drinks a week.

   c. I've had patients mix distilled alcohol with BHB ketones. Not my idea...but it worked. When they felt the need for alcohol, ketones added to distilled drinks seemed to be the least derailing option.

4. **YOU'RE A TYPE-1 DIABETIC AND YOUR AVERAGE BLOOD SUGAR RANGES ABOVE 150.**

5. **YOU'RE A TYPE-2 DIABETIC AND YOUR AVERAGE BLOOD SUGAR SOARS ABOVE 150.**

6. **YOU HAVE INSULIN RESISTANCE OR UNDIAGNOSED DIABETES.**

LET'S START AGAIN

<u>200 Club</u> + <u>DR. CLUB</u> + DAY 4 CLUB

If you are in the 200 Club, or the Dr. Club, or did not pee ketones by Day 4, LET'S START AGAIN.

A slower approach is better for you. Use this two-week countdown.

Two Week Countdown

>   Drink Ketones-In-A-Can
>   Cut sweetness from your drinks
>   No white stuff

BE KETO: USE KETOSIS CHEMISTRY.

Ketosis is not a way of eating. Ketosis is a state of chemistry in your blood. That means you need ketones in circulation. Let me help you. Outsmart or "biohack" that chemistry with supplemental BHB or MCT C8:C10.

If you're struggling by Day 4, supplement your blood with ketones. Drink BHB salts or swallow MCT C8:C10 to forcibly switch your energy. Keep supplementing and checking PeeTones for fourteen days. The presence of ketones will awaken transporters lifting ketones into the new environments. Bridge your body and brain to a new fuel.

Two Week Countdown

Drink Ketones-In-a-Can.

If you are in the Dr. Club or the 200 Club, you will gain the most benefit from sipping on ready-made ketones for 10-14 days. Ketones-In-A-Can prepares the body for the upcoming transition from carb-fuel to fat-fuel.

Much like adding powdered sugar to water, powdered ketones can be mixed into water. Swallow powdered sugar-water for a flash of pine-needle fuel. Swallow ketone-water for longer log-based fuel.

Ketones arrive into your circulation about 15 min after you start drinking them. They remain in circulation for a couple of hours. Ketones (either swallowed or those made by your liver) have two paths out of the body:

1. Burned as fuel in a mitochondria

2. Removed from circulation through the kidney into the urine.

Circulating ketones awaken the cell's parts that use them. Exposure to ketones wakes up the needed cellular parts to transition to nutritional ketosis. Before you take away carbs, add ketones. Buffer the change in your body by sipping ketones before you start cutting carbs. The healthier you are when you begin, the less you need this assistance. Most in the Dr. Club or in the 200 Club have poor health within their cells. This approach delivers keto chemistry to your body and prepares for the removal of carbs.

Sip on them for several hours a day as to constantly add them. Ketones-In-A-Can radically changed the success of insulin-resistant patients' arrival at ketosis. The healthier you get, the less you will need these supplements.

This biohack bridges the transition and helps if you fall off the wagon.

When advising athletes, I use this tip to prepare their bodies too.

BETA-HYDROXYBUTYRATE

Ketogenic chemistry means ketones are in your circulation.

Mix Ketones-in-a-Can with any liquid and drink your keto-chemistry.
Just swallow it.

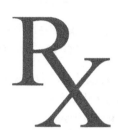

TWICE-DAILY BETA-HYDROXYBUTYRATE.

Twice a day, mix ketones into a drink and sip on them.
The goal is to consume at least 16 grams of ketones over daylight hours.
For two weeks, drink 16 grams of ketones throughout each day.
During those two weeks, lower the number of carbs to as close to 20 as possible.

Keep track of the total carbs while supplementing with Ketones-In-A-Can.
Let Ketones-In-A-Can carry you until you master 20 carbs or less per day.

Be careful NOT TO GUZZLE the drink.
Guzzling ketones turns Ketones-In-A-Can into a laxative. Diarrhea!

Keep checking your PeeTone strips.

Drinking Ketones-In-A-Can saturates the blood with ketones for two to four hours after swallowing it. The science behind the hack starts with circulating ketones.
PeeTones arrive in urine after circulating in the blood for a period of time without getting burned as fuel. The ketones in your urine are leftovers. At first, most cells are not ready to use ketones and many ketones are flushed into the bladder unused.
Rapid consumption of the ketones results in many ketones in your blood, but exposing your cells for a longer portion of the day matters more. SIP ON THEM.

CUT SWEETNESS FROM YOUR DRINKS.

If you failed to make ketones by Day 4, you have something going haywire in the microscopic parts of your cells.

Cut the sweetness out of your drinks— zero carbs, and zero sweeteners in your drinks.

Except for Ketones-In-A-Can, remove all sweet-tasting beverages. I make this exception to allow Ketones-In-A-Can because ... frankly — it works.

The goal is zero calories, zero carbs, and zero sweeteners in your drinks. Start with the removal of all the carbs. Sweeteners should all go too. But for now, the one sweetened drink I allow is Ketones-In-A-Can.

When you take away the sweetness and carbs in your drinks, your tongue will go on strike. Your palate has grown used to that sweet taste. Stop that. With the exception of Ketones-In-A-Can, do your best to remove all sweet-tasting liquids.

Don't advance to the next step until you reset your taste buds away from sweeteners.

Your system will adapt. Give it a chance.

Ketones enter your circulation and deliver more than just fuel. Ketones signal your cells to change the way they work. For the folks reading this section, that cellular advantage matters greatly.

Add fat such as heavy whipping cream, coconut cream, or MCT C8:C10 to that ketone drink. Fat improves the absorption of the ketone salts along with the taste.

We will eventually take away the fat to achieve the ultimate goal of no calories, no carbs, and no sweeteners in the drinks, but that step lies weeks down the road.

NO WHITE STUFF.

During the first week of your your two week countdown, start with no sweets in your drinks except Ketones-In-A-Can. The second week, apply this rule: NO WHITE STUFF.

- No bread.
- No rice.
- No potatoes.
- No pasta.
- No pastries.

Keep that rule for the final 7 consecutive days of your Two Week Countdown. This gives your brain and body space to gently shift chemistry after your cells have seen ketones for the past week. This prevents keto flu. This also prevents the crabbiness on the second and third days that comes with the withdrawal of glucose without ketones.

This Two Week Countdown also gives you time to clean out your cupboards.

ALL OF YOUR CUPBOARDS.

2.6 SETBACKS & STALLS

If you have struggled with your opening week of keto, don't despair. This is not a race. Those who struggle often need keto-chemistry the most. They suffer from longstanding inflammation hidden inside their body. Keto-chemistry reverses inflammation. Continued keto-chemistry repels inflammation from returning.

While you biohack with supplements and slowly reduce the carbs to twenty total carbs per day, consider these tasks.

If you had a setback or stalled in your weight loss, follow these steps:

1. READ YOUR WHY

The first part of this book instructed you to write down your WHY. Re-read that statement. We did that exercise for moments like these.

2. CALL A TOW TRUCK

Support groups are tow trucks. They get people out of the ditch. There's no better time to start a support group than after a fall off the keto wagon. Humility runs high and attracts the right kind of people. Find others trying to improve their health. Join forces. You're not the only one struggling. Look around. Waistlines everywhere stretch to their limit.

Get out of your cubicles, houses, and comfort zones. Look up from the Facebook group and start a real live meeting that meets in person.

Others in your community want to do this too. Be brave. Announce what you are doing. Post the sign-up sheet from Section 1.2 of this workbook. Begin again.

Extend yourself forgiveness and the gentle grace you need. Changing behavior is hard. Inspiration grows in support groups. Setback or stall — be brave enough to try again.

See section 2.9 for details about how to run a group.

3. GRAB THOSE URINE KETONE STICKS.

Testing PeeTones sounds goofy. But this works because it offers personal accountability. Use PeeTones as a plus or minus at this stage of the game. Did you produce ketones? Yes. or No... Keep those ketone strips in your pocket. Use them two or three times a day after a setback.

Ketosis is not a diet; it's chemistry flowing through your veins. Prove to yourself that your chemistry is ketosis. Check!

4. LISTEN TO *ANYWAY YOU CAN*

If you fell off the wagon, listen to the audiobook *A*. This is the first book I wrote. It is truly a gift from God. I shared a story about my mom and the lessons that I wrote down for her. Those lessons rescued her during this critical phase of her life. The story reminds the listener of how many ways ketones help out an old chemistry set. The compassionate story helps you root for the underdog, Grandma Rose. You will finish the book inspired and willing to try again.

5. RETURN TO CRONOMETER

Remember the app I asked you to download at the beginning. Find that. Start over. Take an honest count of your carbs again. Be real. Don't round down.

Instead of slamming your total carbs to 20, let's step down a bit slower. Cut your carbs by 'some.' Use your tracking tool to see if you kept the number steady for 5 straight days. Then cut the number again.

Stay there for a week. This shift isn't as dramatic to your system. It allows time. Time to assess your relationship with different carbs. That sounds weird, "Relationship with food." During these steps, notice which foods trigger you the most. Which carbs do you "make room" for? What food pulls the strongest on your desire? Track to see if you stayed out of the ditch for a whole week with your newly reduced carbs. With this success, you can set another minor yet measurable goal.

6. BIOHACK WITH <u>BHB.</u>

If you fell off the wagon and you dread the effort of transitioning again, HACK IT.
This time, let me help you, chemically.
Do the 14 Day BHB Challenge outlined in the last section. For 14 days, sip on Ketones-In-A-Can.

Carbohydrates won your first round. Temptation conquered your brain. This time around, we'll fight those carbohydrates with a little more chemistry and a slower transition. Work on reducing those carbs while drinking ketones.

When folks get stuck in a season of temptation, a bottle of Ketones-In-A-Can rescues them. When snacking derails the afternoon or evening, sip on BHB to suppress hunger, satisfy cravings, and bridge through the struggle. BHB boosts you out of the ditch.

2.7 Day 5: Magnesium

Fill out this chart on your fifth day.

Time	Blood Pressure	Heart Rate	PeeTone Strip Color	Total Carbs	Bowel Activity
			0 1 2 3 4 5 6		
			0 1 2 3 4 5 6		
			0 1 2 3 4 5 6		
			0 1 2 3 4 5 6		
			0 1 2 3 4 5 6		
			0 1 2 3 4 5 6		
			0 1 2 3 4 5 6		
			0 1 2 3 4 5 6		
			0 1 2 3 4 5 6		
			0 1 2 3 4 5 6		
			0 1 2 3 4 5 6		
			0 1 2 3 4 5 6		
			0 1 2 3 4 5 6		
			0 1 2 3 4 5 6		
			0 1 2 3 4 5 6		
			0 1 2 3 4 5 6		
			0 1 2 3 4 5 6		
			0 1 2 3 4 5 6		

REPLACE MAGNESIUM

1. MOM

Milk of Magnesia is an over-the-counter medication. In the first weeks of keto, one of the most common minerals lost is magnesium. This magnesium-filled liquid medication helps replenish your missing magnesium. I guarantee it has magnesium in it. Swallow a big swig. Thirty minutes later the gurgles in your tummy followed by diarrhea prove you chugged magnesium. Flushing most of it down the toilet isn't the plan. Instead of a gulp, add a tablespoon to the water you drink. Sip magnesium-spiked water all day long. This will certainly increase the magnesium in your body. It is cheap, easy to find, and safe.

2. USE YOUR USE SKIN: EPSOM SALT BATH

Pour that full 5-pound bag of magnesium salt (Epsom salt) into the bathtub. Set the timer for 40 minutes. Fill with warm water and sit.

Sit for at least 40 minutes with the warm, salted water up to your armpits.

Keep the water warm with a trickle of heat coming into the tub for the full 40 minutes.

Magnesium is one of those salts flushing out of your kidney. You can't feel it...yet.

3. USE YOUR SKIN: FLOAT SPA

This is the best. This is a maximum Epsom salt bath. Floatation tanks add 1500 pounds of Epsom salt to a single-person pod. Much like the Dead Sea, the salinity of the water is so high, you can't sink. Enter into your private pod wearing your birthday suit. Close the cover to your pod for a vacation wrapped inside an hour. You don't have to close the cover, but I love it.

Time-out. No light. No sound. Floating in warm water. Suspended without touch, light or noise.

All sensory input stops. My mind floats into relaxation mode.

4. OTHER MAGNESIUM SUPPLEMENTS

TAKE A SUPPLEMENT: Names of replacement supplements include magnesium citrate, magnesium chloride, magnesium hydroxylate, and magnesium glycinate. Magnesium glycinate and Slow-Mag (a slow-digesting form of magnesium chloride) tends to cause fewer loose stools or other digestive problems.

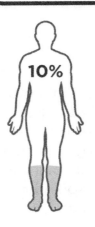

EPSOM FOOT SOAK:

Surface area = 10%

Concentration = 10 pounds

Time = 60 minutes

0.1 x 10 x 60 = 60

2 five-pound bags (12 cups)
of Epsom salt in foot basin

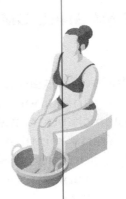

MAGNESIUM FORMULA

The mathematical formula for delivering magnewsium through the skin:
**The conentration of magnesium X the surface area of your
skin exposed to magnesium X time.**

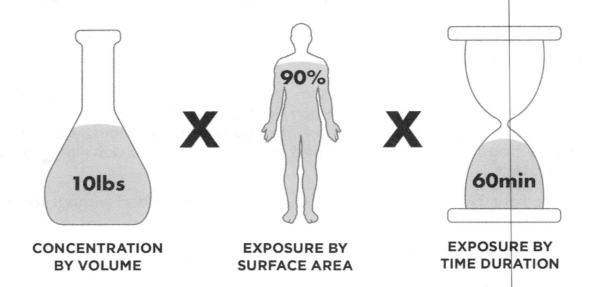

CONCENTRATION BY VOLUME	EXPOSURE BY SURFACE AREA	EXPOSURE BY TIME DURATION
10lbs	90%	60min

Notice the dynamic impact the different scenarios delivered. The small surface area of skin touching the water in the foot soak delivers much less magnesium than the salted baths. In comparison, the Float Spa offers such high salinity that it forces you to float. When adding the greatest surface area to the supersaturated water, the impact on magnesium replacement far exceeds the other options.

ketoCONTINUUM Workbook

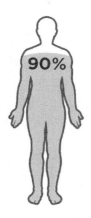

EPSOM SALT BATH:
Surface area = 90%
Concentration = 5 pounds
Time = 60 minutes
0.9 x 5 x 60 = 270
5 pounds of salt = 270

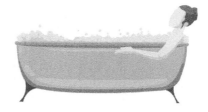

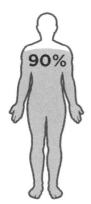

EPSOM SALT BATH:
Surface area = 90%
Concentration = 10 pounds
Time = 60 minutes
0.9 x 10 x 60 = 540
10 pounds of salt = 540

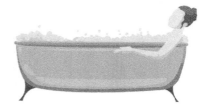

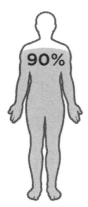

FLOAT SPA:
Surface area = 90%
Concentration = 1,500 pounds
Time = 60 minutes
0.9 x 1500 x 60 = 81,000

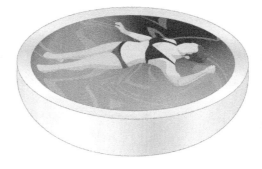

Magnesium Shortage Symptoms Chart

	Week 1	Week 2	Week 3
# Magnesium Soaks/Baths in Past Week	1 2 3 4 5 6 7	1 2 3 4 5 6 7	1 2 3 4 5 6 7
Days You Swallowed Magnesium Supplements	1 2 3 4 5 6 7	1 2 3 4 5 6 7	1 2 3 4 5 6 7
Energy	HIGH Medium Low	HIGH Medium Low	HIGH Medium Low
Concentration	FOCUSED Distracted	FOCUSED Distracted	FOCUSED Distracted
Motivation	MOTIVATED Unmotivated	MOTIVATED Unmotivated	MOTIVATED Unmotivated
Days of Bowel Movement	1 2 3 4 5 6 7	1 2 3 4 5 6 7	1 2 3 4 5 6 7
Muscle Cramps	NO CRAMPS Cramps	NO CRAMPS Cramps	NO CRAMPS Cramps
Headaches	NO PAIN Headaches	NO PAIN Headaches	NO PAIN Headaches
Back Pain (muscle)	NO PAIN Back Pain	NO PAIN Back Pain	NO PAIN Back Pain
Neck Pain (muscle)	NO PAIN Neck Pain	NO PAIN Neck Pain	NO PAIN Neck Pain
Tremor	NO TREMOR Trembling	NO TREMOR Trembling	NO TREMOR Trembling
Mood (Depression)	NONE Depressed	NONE Depressed	NONE Depressed
Mood (Worried)	NONE Worried	NONE Worried	NONE Worried
Memory	NORMAL Forgetful	NORMAL Forgetful	NORMAL Forgetful
Brain Fog	NONE Foggy	NONE Foggy	NONE Foggy
Mood (Grouchy)	NONE Grouchy	NONE Grouchy	NONE Grouchy

ketoCONTINUUM Workbook

2.8 Day 6: Calories & Cravings

Fill out this chart on your sixth day.

Time	Blood Pressure	Heart Rate	PeeTone Strip Color	Total Carbs	Bowel Activity
			0 1 2 3 4 5 6		
			0 1 2 3 4 5 6		
			0 1 2 3 4 5 6		
			0 1 2 3 4 5 6		
			0 1 2 3 4 5 6		
			0 1 2 3 4 5 6		
			0 1 2 3 4 5 6		
			0 1 2 3 4 5 6		
			0 1 2 3 4 5 6		
			0 1 2 3 4 5 6		
			0 1 2 3 4 5 6		
			0 1 2 3 4 5 6		
			0 1 2 3 4 5 6		
			0 1 2 3 4 5 6		
			0 1 2 3 4 5 6		
			0 1 2 3 4 5 6		
			0 1 2 3 4 5 6		

WHY COUNT CALORIES WHEN YOUR BODY DOESN'T

CALORIES: no receptor in your body keeps track of calories

CHEMISTRY BEFORE CALORIES

EAT FAT. Track your intake with Cronometer App. Keep your total carbs under 20 and your fat intake high. That's how you surge hormones and reset your chemistry.

CALORIES MATTER AFTER THE BODY HAS BEEN KETO-ADAPTED.

- Track total carbs first. Become keto-adapted. Don't pay attention to calories until you are keto-adapted.

- During the first weeks of ketosis, learn to listen to your body. Most can barely 'hear' the whisper from their fat-built hormones.

- Chewing and swallowing carbs ORDERS your body to make insulin. Your body will faithfully follow your chemical orders. It will store food

- Address your body's chemistry first. The chemistry outranks calories when you first begin a ketogenic diet.

- Change your metabolism and cut down insulin production.

- Turn down your insulin spigot when you consume fat instead of carbs.

EAT ONLY WHEN YOU ARE HUNGRY. LISTEN FOR HUNGER.

- The sensation of hunger comes from one HORMONE

- The satiated feeling comes from the OPPOSITE HORMONE

- True hunger arrives slowly (over a 30 minute time) and leaves slowly (15 minutes).

CRAVINGS = NO FAT-BASED HORMONES.

- Cravings punch you in the nose when they hit. Beware. Even the no-calorie sweeteners, like stevia and erythritol, light up a brain scan with cravings. Tickling those nerves with fake sugars = danger.

HABITS = AUTOMATIC.

- Change the pattern to break mindless habits.
  - o Example: Enter the house so you don't walk through the kitchen.
  - o Example: Instead of dessert, play a game of cribbage as a way to spend more time together around the table. Leave out the food.

- Empty the cupboard that keeps your snacks. Put the box in the garage.

CRAVING ANALYSIS EXERCISE

Here is a 10-minute exercise to understand your food cravings.

Place food that you love in front of you—or somehow induce a food craving. Or wait for the next one to arrive. Notice your "desire" for sweetness before you start the experiment. Mark the desired column 1-5 as to how much desire you have for the food. One = No desire. Five is INTENSE desire. Set a timer for 10 min. Every 30 seconds, re-rank your desire for the food. Don't eat any food.

Use the next charts to document your craving. This WORKS. You must document it for it to work. Use this more than once with a variety of food.

Once you have several cravings documented, be sure to do the follow-up exercise.

EMOTIONS

Cravings are often linked to an emotion. This Craving-Analysis exercise helps you slow down the moment and study it. When I do this exercise with patients, they often want to ignore their emotions by labeling it boredom or simply stating, "feel nothing." If we persist in the moment, they unlock an understanding of their feelings. As you hold your thoughts in the craving moment, look through these sections of words. Find what emotion you are feeling. I have listed the words of protective feelings, also called negative emotions. The list of feelings often coaxes patients into that moment of craving food. Suppressing the negative feeling by eating food has been a default coping skill to many patients for years. Notice why you eat. What feelings do you associate with eating? Is it hunger? Do you actually feel hungry when you eat?

ANGER

Annoyed, agitated, fed up, frustrated, irritated, mad, critical, resentful, disgusted, outraged, raging, furious seething, livid, bitter

DEPRESSED

Lousy, disappointed, discouraged, ashamed, powerless, diminished, guilty, dissatisfied, miserable, detestable, pungent, despicable, disgusting, abominable terrible, in despair, sulky, bad, a sense of loss

FEAR

Timid, uneasy, tense, nervous, insecure, cowardly, worried, afraid, threatened, frightened, intimidated, fearful, anxious, panicked, horrified, terrified, cowardly, quaking, menaced, wary

PANIC

Mixed up, unsure, uncomfortable, troubled, perplexed, insecure, disoriented, stunned, shocked, rattled, stuck, lost, trapped, desperate, helpless, frozen, hysterical, paralyzed

HURT

Crushed, tormented, deprived, pained, tortured, dejected, rejected, injured, offended, afflicted, aching, victimized, heartbroken, agonized, appalled, humiliated, wronged, alienated

HELPLESS

Incapable, alone, paralyzed, fatigued, useless, inferior, vulnerable, empty, forced, hesitant, despair, frustrated, distressed, woeful, pathetic, dominated

SAD

Tearful, sorrowful, pained, grief, anguish, desolate, desperate, pessimistic, unhappy, lonely, mournful, dismayed

10-MINUTE FOOD CRAVING EXERCISE

Document which food you're craving. Then set the clock for 10 minutes. As it counts down, fill in the line every 30 seconds. Cursive writing connects to a deeper section of your subconscience. After several sessions a pattern emerges. If you can't see the pattern, consider sharing this with a friend of advisor.

Which food are you craving?								
Date	Time	Salt Crystal	Desire Level					Notes: What else is on your mind? What is going on around you? Which emotion do you feel?
	Start	Yes / No	1	2	3	4	5	
	0:30 sec	Yes / No	1	2	3	4	5	
	1:00	Yes / No	1	2	3	4	5	
	1:30	Yes / No	1	2	3	4	5	
	2:00	Yes / No	1	2	3	4	5	
	2:30	Yes / No	1	2	3	4	5	
	3:00	Yes / No	1	2	3	4	5	
	3:30	Yes / No	1	2	3	4	5	
	4:00	Yes / No	1	2	3	4	5	
	4:30	Yes / No	1	2	3	4	5	
	5:00	Yes / No	1	2	3	4	5	
	5:30	Yes / No	1	2	3	4	5	
	6:00	Yes / No	1	2	3	4	5	
	6:30	Yes / No	1	2	3	4	5	
	7:00	Yes / No	1	2	3	4	5	
	7:30	Yes / No	1	2	3	4	5	
	8:00	Yes / No	1	2	3	4	5	
	8:30	Yes / No	1	2	3	4	5	
	9:00	Yes / No	1	2	3	4	5	
	9:30	Yes / No	1	2	3	4	5	
	10:00	Yes / No	1	2	3	4	5	

Each time you do a 10-minute Food Craving Exercise, use this chart to analyze your thoughts. After several entries, look for patterns.

Date	What time of day did it happen?	Emotions Associated		How long did the sensation last?		What made it go away?	
		CRAVING	HUNGER	CRAVING	HUNGER	CRAVING	HUNGER
		YES	NO	<5 MIN	>15 MIN	• Meditation singing • Splash water to your face • Salt to your tongue • Go for a walk	Time
		YES	NO	<5 MIN	>15 MIN		Time
		YES	NO	<5 MIN	>15 MIN		Time
		YES	NO	<5 MIN	>15 MIN		Time
		YES	NO	<5 MIN	>15 MIN		Time
		YES	NO	<5 MIN	>15 MIN		Time
		YES	NO	<5 MIN	>15 MIN		Time
		YES	NO	<5 MIN	>15 MIN		Time
		YES	NO	<5 MIN	>15 MIN		Time
		YES	NO	<5 MIN	>15 MIN		Time

10-MINUTE FOOD CRAVING EXERCISE

Which food are you craving?								
Date	Time	Salt Crystal	Desire Level					Notes: What else is on your mind? What is going on around you? Which emotion do you feel?
	Start	Yes / No	1	2	3	4	5	
	0:30 sec	Yes / No	1	2	3	4	5	
	1:00	Yes / No	1	2	3	4	5	
	1:30	Yes / No	1	2	3	4	5	
	2:00	Yes / No	1	2	3	4	5	
	2:30	Yes / No	1	2	3	4	5	
	3:00	Yes / No	1	2	3	4	5	
	3:30	Yes / No	1	2	3	4	5	
	4:00	Yes / No	1	2	3	4	5	
	4:30	Yes / No	1	2	3	4	5	
	5:00	Yes / No	1	2	3	4	5	
	5:30	Yes / No	1	2	3	4	5	
	6:00	Yes / No	1	2	3	4	5	
	6:30	Yes / No	1	2	3	4	5	
	7:00	Yes / No	1	2	3	4	5	
	7:30	Yes / No	1	2	3	4	5	
	8:00	Yes / No	1	2	3	4	5	
	8:30	Yes / No	1	2	3	4	5	
	9:00	Yes / No	1	2	3	4	5	
	9:30	Yes / No	1	2	3	4	5	
	10:00	Yes / No	1	2	3	4	5	

10-MINUTE FOOD CRAVING EXERCISE

Which food are you craving?								
Date	**Time**	**Salt Crystal**	**Desire Level**					**Notes:** What else is on your mind? What is going on around you? Which emotion do you feel?
	Start	Yes / No	1	2	3	4	5	
	0:30 sec	Yes / No	1	2	3	4	5	
	1:00	Yes / No	1	2	3	4	5	
	1:30	Yes / No	1	2	3	4	5	
	2:00	Yes / No	1	2	3	4	5	
	2:30	Yes / No	1	2	3	4	5	
	3:00	Yes / No	1	2	3	4	5	
	3:30	Yes / No	1	2	3	4	5	
	4:00	Yes / No	1	2	3	4	5	
	4:30	Yes / No	1	2	3	4	5	
	5:00	Yes / No	1	2	3	4	5	
	5:30	Yes / No	1	2	3	4	5	
	6:00	Yes / No	1	2	3	4	5	
	6:30	Yes / No	1	2	3	4	5	
	7:00	Yes / No	1	2	3	4	5	
	7:30	Yes / No	1	2	3	4	5	
	8:00	Yes / No	1	2	3	4	5	
	8:30	Yes / No	1	2	3	4	5	
	9:00	Yes / No	1	2	3	4	5	
	9:30	Yes / No	1	2	3	4	5	
	10:00	Yes / No	1	2	3	4	5	

10-MINUTE FOOD CRAVING EXERCISE

Which food are you craving?								
Date	**Time**	**Salt Crystal**	**Desire Level**					**Notes:** **What else is on your mind? What is going on around you?** **Which emotion do you feel?**
	Start	Yes / No	1	2	3	4	5	
	0:30 sec	Yes / No	1	2	3	4	5	
	1:00	Yes / No	1	2	3	4	5	
	1:30	Yes / No	1	2	3	4	5	
	2:00	Yes / No	1	2	3	4	5	
	2:30	Yes / No	1	2	3	4	5	
	3:00	Yes / No	1	2	3	4	5	
	3:30	Yes / No	1	2	3	4	5	
	4:00	Yes / No	1	2	3	4	5	
	4:30	Yes / No	1	2	3	4	5	
	5:00	Yes / No	1	2	3	4	5	
	5:30	Yes / No	1	2	3	4	5	
	6:00	Yes / No	1	2	3	4	5	
	6:30	Yes / No	1	2	3	4	5	
	7:00	Yes / No	1	2	3	4	5	
	7:30	Yes / No	1	2	3	4	5	
	8:00	Yes / No	1	2	3	4	5	
	8:30	Yes / No	1	2	3	4	5	
	9:00	Yes / No	1	2	3	4	5	
	9:30	Yes / No	1	2	3	4	5	
	10:00	Yes / No	1	2	3	4	5	

10-MINUTE FOOD CRAVING EXERCISE

Which food are you craving?								
Date	**Time**	**Salt Crystal**	**Desire Level**					**Notes:** What else is on your mind? What is going on around you? Which emotion do you feel?
	Start	Yes / No	1	2	3	4	5	
	0.30 sec	Yes / No	1	2	3	4	5	
	1:00	Yes / No	1	2	3	4	5	
	1:30	Yes / No	1	2	3	4	5	
	2:00	Yes / No	1	2	3	4	5	
	2:30	Yes / No	1	2	3	4	5	
	3:00	Yes / No	1	2	3	4	5	
	3:30	Yes / No	1	2	3	4	5	
	4:00	Yes / No	1	2	3	4	5	
	4:30	Yes / No	1	2	3	4	5	
	5:00	Yes / No	1	2	3	4	5	
	5:30	Yes / No	1	2	3	4	5	
	6:00	Yes / No	1	2	3	4	5	
	6:30	Yes / No	1	2	3	4	5	
	7:00	Yes / No	1	2	3	4	5	
	7:30	Yes / No	1	2	3	4	5	
	8:00	Yes / No	1	2	3	4	5	
	8:30	Yes / No	1	2	3	4	5	
	9:00	Yes / No	1	2	3	4	5	
	9:30	Yes / No	1	2	3	4	5	
	10:00	Yes / No	1	2	3	4	5	

Now look back at several of your moments where you desired food. Do you notice a pattern? A theme?

Write down what is similar about these situations. Consider time, place, people, emotions, and level of fatigue.

ketoCONTINUUM **Workbook**

In the end, it doesn't matter if it is a craving or a pang of real hunger. The exercise teaches what your enemy looks and feels like. You must learn how to get through the moment. Study why you desire food. You will learn much about yourself as you do this exercise. Once you begin to process why you are thinking about food, embrace the discomfort. If it is a craving, it will pass. If it is hunger, it will pass too. Push through the moment. Salt through the moment. Use the exercise to study yourself.

Personally, I have learned to write down my prayers of gratitude during times of cravings. Using long-hand cursive slows down my thinking and keeps me focused on the many things for which I am grateful. There is advanced neuroscience at work in this exercise. You can only gain that benefit by doing the exercise over and over.

LEFT-HANDED LOOPS

Get a pencil. Place it in your NON-dominate hand. [If right-handed, use your left hand. If left-handed, use your right hand.]

Set a timer for THREE MINUTES. When you start the timer, use your non-dominate hand to write cursive lower-case l's across the page. Keep writing cursive l's for the full three minutes. Do not speak. Do not make noise of any sort. Do not look at the clock.

Just write cursive l's for three minutes.

After the exercise, assess the intensity of your craving.

This "Left-Handed Loop" exercise is a form of meditation. Use this bio-hack to abort the negative repetitive thoughts when they start circling in your mind. I have used this technique in thousands of patients. It is an effective beginning point to learn how to meditate your way out of repeating, sabotaging thoughts.

Patients will present with pages upon pages of left-handed loops. As they practice this rhythmical writing exercise with their non-dominant hand, their body, brain, and spirit grow calmer.

ketoCONTINUUM Workbook

2.9 MEETINGS & MIRROR NEURONS

If you skipped these steps earlier...now is the time to try again. Do this.

1. Write this signup

    a. Write down these words: "I am starting a keto support group to improve my health. Join me, please. Every Tuesday at 3:30 - 4:30 PM in the conference room. Starts in August. Will continue through October and then re-assess. Please come."

    b. Handwritten signs work better than printed ones. Consider adding tear-offs along the bottom with the time and address. Notice your commitment lasts for three months. Once this sign-up hangs on a wall for others to read, you have accountability.

2. Focus on Who

    a. Focus on attracting people, not the location. Write down five places you interact with people. (See section 1.2.) Consider the office, church, the kids' school activities, and volunteer groups.

    b. Write down five people that you could reach out to in a moment of struggle. When tragedy or sadness hits your life, who would call? Write down their names. (See section 1.2)

3. Post the signup at your 5 locations. Hand the signup to your 5 people. Look them in the eye and say these words, "Please come. I could use some support."

4. Select a Location: Must be convenient for you, the leader. Not too convenient...but convenient enough to keep you consistent. If you're sitting alone at your kitchen table calling it a keto support meeting, you made it too convenient for you. Municipalities have public rooms. Reserve a room for 3 months as described in your signup. Here are some ideas of municipalities in your area.

    • Schools
    • Libraries
    • Community Centers/Rooms
    • Churches
    • Conference Rooms (ask your employer if you can borrow one)

5. Weekly: You must hold meetings weekly. It doesn't matter if no one shows up for the first several. You are doing this to set a pattern for YOU.

6. Keep it FREE

   a. A free meeting decreases the barrier to entrance. This really helps those people walking through the door— whether it is their first time or after a setback.

   b. Attracts people who want to change. Sales experts will tell you that if you want people to commit, charge them money. There is truth to that statement, but I find the culture of genuine change grows best when you cut the strings of manipulating people's behavior and offer them your example. Your actions will fire their mirror neurons and you will both be better because of it.

7. Use these best practices for meetings:

   a. Start each meeting promptly. Arrive a few minutes early. Set up the room to promote eye contact between attendees by placing the chairs in a circle or around a table.

   b. Stop when you say you will stop. This sends a subconscious message to your attendees to show up on time and that you won't steal their time by extending a meeting longer than stated.

   c. Anonymity and confidentiality are required. Share the education you learn at keto-group without sharing identity.

   d. Do not gossip. Talk about yourself. Not others. Instead of advising others, share personal stories with similar struggles.

   e. Share your own thoughts and feelings. Sharing improves a group. Advising divides a group. Let their mirror neurons connect the dots.

   f. No cross-talk. A separate conversation with your neighbor limits sharing. Bring forth your comments in a way that all can hear and participate.

   g. VETERANS: Check in first. Lead with your example and show newbies the culture of the group. Trigger their mirror neurons.

   h. NEWBIES: Instruct newbies to watch for the first couple of meetings. Encourage them to observe the veterans and follow their examples—usually, that means at least one meeting.

   i. Don't share recipes at keto-group. This sounds like a safe idea, but quickly gets hijacked by folks struggling with food addiction. Stay on the behavior and activities that have replaced eating.

8. Don't allow food at keto group: Much like no alcohol is allowed at an AA meeting, no food is allowed at keto group.

PURPOSE OF MEETINGS

1. **To connect—not to educate**

    a. Keep your focus on relationships and human connections. This decreases the burden on the leadership & provides the most important reason for a group: SUPPORT. Show your example—even when it's flawed.

    b. LEADERSHIP - BE SURE TO LEAD!

       i. Leadership should lead the way by sharing first. This provides a prototype for others in the group to follow.

       ii. Mirror Neurons: Politely announce that newcomers are to watch. We will do their introductions at the end. Newcomers can quickly take over a meeting and derail the community of support. Their eager energy can siphon all the focus into one person. They will get support. Their first role is to observe. Veterans check-in first. Offer veterans the center stage to share the best part of their past week and one struggle. Discussions can slide off-topic yet still prove relevant. Struggles with food frequently arise from stressors in life. Allow the topic to drift towards those stressors. Bring the conversations back on topic if the focus goes too far.

       iii. Leadership - It is your job to stop cross-talk when that happens. If 2 people begin a side conversation while someone else is sharing, politely say these words, "Please hold that conversation for everyone to hear." Years of running small groups taught me this skill. Use my pain. Stop crosstalk during a meeting.

       iv. Leadership - It is your job to not let one person (especially a newbie) take over your meeting. Politely do your job, "I appreciate your enthusiasm, but I'd like you to watch a bit longer before offering your testimony / questions."

       v. Leadership - Help attendees stay focused on their own experiences and choices. If you see this happening, use the teachable moment. Consider saying this, "Instead of telling Mrs. Smith what to do, could you rephrase your comment. Share with the group how you have had a similar experience and what you did in that situation."

2. **Extend grace**. Grace = a disposition of kindness and compassion. People will return if they feel the presence of grace. Practice spreading grace. We all need a little more of this.

   a. When listening to the struggles of others, think about this word: GRACE. A culture of grace grows through example. Fill the meetings with words of forgiveness when you screw it up. Show one another how to start over, and keep trying.

   b. When you fail, extend grace to yourself. When others fail or struggle, do the same. This creates a very welcoming environment for learning how to change behavior.

3. **Curriculum**

   a. Do not create this yourself. That is too much for the leader. Stay focused on relationships. Leave the content to experts.

   b. TOPIC IDEAS:

   - HI/LO check-in. HI: Share a keto-success of your week. LO: Share a keto disappointment from the week.

   - Share your KETO WHY

   - Check-in with your current status on the ketoCONTINUUM. Photocopy the chart on the next page along with the Check-In cards. These tools help folks assess themselves.

   - Offer your examples of times when you said, "NO" to temptations.

   - Share a cravings analysis exercise.

   - Identify and share a coping skills you are working on

   - Share a personal tactic on how to avoid carbs. Share the fridge sign found at the end of this section.

   - Set a goal for the upcoming week.

   - If you have a quiet group, watch a short video from Consistently Keto or of the playlist All Things Keto. Share a comment about what you learned.

     ☺ Click play at the beginning of the meeting and watch it together if the video is short. Another approach is to assign the videos as the pre-group preparation. Watching the video before the group provides an excellent foundation for discussion. It does take more planning and engaged participants to pull that off.

     ☺ If no one shows up, just push play. Know that the persistence of a meeting will attract people. Stay the course, don't give up.

ketoCONTINUUM ROADMAP

	ketoCONTINUUM	WHO DOES THE WORK?	TEST	GUIDELINES	NEXT STEPS	
BEGINNER	**#1:** I eat every 2-4 hours	CHEMISTRY CARRIES YOU	X	Fueled on glucose. Must refuel often. Never fueled by ketones.		**4-6 WEEKS**
	#2: I eat every 6-8 hours LESS THAN 20 total carbs		Urine PeeTone Strips	Eat <20 total carbs per day. Ketosis begins. Fat-based hormones rise. Eating happens less frequently.	Be sure to eat high fat with low carbs. Your body uses the fat to restore your fat built hormones. Elevated insulin within your body prevents you from using the stored fat. You must eat the fat.	
	#3: I "accidentally" missed a meal. [Keto-adapted]			Fat supplies the resources needed to make fat-built hormones approach healthy levels. Appetite decreases according to body's chemistry.	Sometimes it takes 10 weeks before this moment happens. Don't look at the scale. Listen for absence of hunger.	
BASELINE METABOLISM	**#4:** Eat 2 meals per day	YOU DO THE WORK. Discipline needed for each new step.		Choose to eat only 2 meals per day.	Succeed 7 days in a row before advancing.	**LIVE HERE**
	#5: 16:8			Eat ALL food, snacks and supplements in an 8-hour window. No eating, snacking or chewing for 16 hours.	That means no gum during fasting hours. Suck on salt if you need a substitute. Keep your coffee filled with fat.	
	#6: Advanced 16:8			Clean up your morning drink. Remove all calories and sweeteners. Morning drink = no fat, no MCT, no butter, no sweeteners, no calories. The 16 hours = only salt, water, black coffee or tea.	Don't remove the fat from your morning drink before this phase. You needed it to get here. Now it's time to let it go.	
	#7: 23:1 OMAD ALL in one hour		Blood Ketone Strips	ALL calories and sweeteners in one hour. 23 hours = Only salt, water, tea or coffee.	Begin checking blood numbers right before you eat.	
	#8: Advanced 23:1/OMAD			Move eating-hour within 11 hours following sunrise to match your circadian rhythm.	Record the Dr. Boz ratio first thing in the morning. Repeat before eating.	
STRESSING METABOLISM	**#9:** 36-hour fast	PSYCHOLOGY. Use tribe for best results.		Fast for 36 hours. No calories. No sweeteners. Start in evening as to use 2 cycles of sleep during the 36 hours.	Begin fast after evening meal. DANGER: If on blood pressure meds or blood sugar lowering meds. ASK YOUR DOCTOR.	**USE INTERMITTENTLY**
	#10: 36-hour fast without a celebration meal			After 36-hour fast, return to your normal pattern of eating without a splurge meal.	Offer a group fasting routine to others in your tribe. Fast together.	
	#11: 48-hour fast			Fast for 48 hours. No calories. No sweeteners.	Safe to try twice a week. Unlike the 36-hour fast, this option keeps meals at the same time each day.	
	#12: 72-hour fast			Fast for 72 hours. No calories. No sweeteners.	When the timing is right, stress your metabolism with 8 weeks of a 72-hour fast. The rest of the week, return to your BASELINE METABOLISM. The best transitions happen through this challenge.	

ketoCONTINUUM Check-In Cards

#1 I eat every 2–4 hours	#7 23:1 OMAD: ALL in one hour. 23 hours=No calories or sweeteners.
#2 LESS THAN 20 total carbs. I eat every 6–8 hours.	#8 Advanced 23:1/OMAD. Your 1 hour of eating happens within the 11 hours following sunrise.
#3 I "accidentally" missed a meal. [Keto-adapted]	
#4 Eat 2 meals per day.	#9 36-hour fast
#5 16:8 ALL food, snacks, and supplements in an 8-hour window.	#10 36-hour fast without a celebration meal
#6 Advanced 16:8 Clean up morning drink. No calories or sweetener in AM drink.	#11 48-hour fast
	#12 72-hour fast

#1 I eat every 2–4 hours	#7 23:1 OMAD: ALL in one hour. 23 hours=No calories or sweeteners.
#2 LESS THAN 20 total carbs. I eat every 6–8 hours.	#8 Advanced 23:1/OMAD. Your 1 hour of eating happens within the 11 hours following sunrise.
#3 I "accidentally" missed a meal. [Keto-adapted]	
#4 Eat 2 meals per day.	#9 36-hour fast
#5 16:8 ALL food, snacks, and supplements in an 8-hour window.	#10 36-hour fast without a celebration meal
#6 Advanced 16:8 Clean up morning drink. No calories or sweetener in AM drink.	#11 48-hour fast
	#12 72-hour fast

#1 I eat every 2–4 hours	#7 23:1 OMAD: ALL in one hour. 23 hours=No calories or sweeteners.
#2 LESS THAN 20 total carbs. I eat every 6–8 hours.	#8 Advanced 23:1/OMAD. Your 1 hour of eating happens within the 11 hours following sunrise.
#3 I "accidentally" missed a meal. [Keto-adapted]	
#4 Eat 2 meals per day.	#9 36-hour fast
#5 16:8 ALL food, snacks, and supplements in an 8-hour window.	#10 36-hour fast without a celebration meal
#6 Advanced 16:8 Clean up morning drink. No calories or sweetener in AM drink.	#11 48-hour fast
	#12 72-hour fast

4. **Accountability Partner**
    a. FIND ONE. Start by looking for others who attend keto-group. The tough phase is around the corner and accountability partners make a huge difference. Example: "I need an accountability partner for 6 weeks. My goal is to get through ketoCONTINUUM #4 in 6 weeks."
    b. Set time commitments with boundaries with accountability partners:
        • Agree to be partners for 6 weeks. You can extend the time, but you also can bow out if the timing are not working.
        • Check-in once a week by phone.
        • Share your 6-week goal. Both of you.

You're not married to your accountability partner. This is a literal statement and a figurative one. Don't ask your spouse to be your accountability partner. Although this pair-up happens, the best results link you to a person that is not in your house or dwelling. This makes the "break up" normal — not awkward. Don't be surprised if it takes a few tries to find the right person and the timing for both of you.

5. **Mirror Neurons** Activate mirror neurons during group.
    a. Come to the meeting and share your journey. Share your struggles. This type of education rewires your brain through your MIRROR NEURONS.
    b. Watch group members struggle. You learn.
    c. Watch them succeed. You learn.
    d. Watch them encourage one another. You learn.

6. Help Others through the First Failure Many people fail on the keto diet between weeks 2-4. Creating a culture of support helps the leader stay the course, and helps members return to keto chemistry as quickly as possible. Side-step common mistakes by preparing.
    a. Drink lots of salted fluid before eating.
    b. Salt sucking works. It sounds so strange, but it really helps. I shake my head and laugh as I type this, but it has course-corrected many lost Neurons.
    c. Plan your first meeting. Be brave. Post the signup.
    d. Say, "NO!" To OMAD (One Meal A Day.) It is not time yet. WARNING: If you make this dietary change at the wrong time, you're VERY likely to fail and fall backward!
    e. Escape through the Audiobook *Anyway You Can* or watch the YouTube Documentary: American Traddiction: Breaking Carb Addiction

FRIDGE SIGN

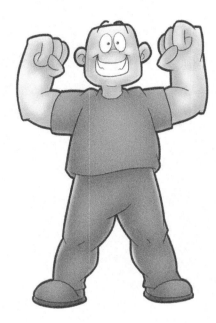

You are NOT hungry.
You are bored.

SHUT THE DOOR.

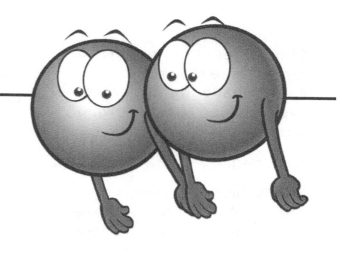

ketoCONTINUUM

SECTION

3

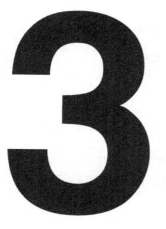

BECOMING KETO ADAPTED

3.1   Week 2 Challenges

3.2   ketoCONTINUUM #3

3.3   ketoCONTINUUM #4

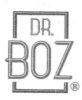

BozMD.com

3.1 WEEK 2 CHALLENGES

Challenges are meant to repeat more than once.
Each challenge is better explained on the following pages.

First, begin.

This sounds obvious, right? The skills found in these challenges better prepare you for the next section. When patients fail at the advancing levels, I often review this chart with them. Many times this chart is blank. Learn these skills by doing them.

Next, mark the date you succeed the FIRST time with each challenge.

Use the other columns for the repeats of each challenge. And document the date of the subsequent successful challenges.

Day: Challenge	1st Success
DAY 8: Consume only calorie-free unsweetened drinks.	
DAY 9: Eat a can of sardines.	
DAY 10: Identify your accountability partner.	
DAY 11: Take a magnesium bath or float.	
DAY 12: Conduct a craving analysis exercise. [Chart found in Section 2.8]	
DAY 13: Watch the sleep lecture. Fill out the sleep chart.	
DAY 14: Test your social strength.	

2nd Success	3rd Success	4th Success

CHALLENGE FOR DAY 8:

1. At least ONE drink with NO calories or sweeteners. The goal is NO sweet drinks and no calories. Keep drinks boring. Frame it this way: if you get your joy from added flavor in a drink, assess your life. Find a volunteer habit. Seek to do an act of kindness for one stranger per day. At first, it may feel stressful, but soon your soul will fill with joy when you do it. Trust me, it is WAY more pleasure than a flavored drink.

   Examples:
   - Water
   - Coffee (black)
   - Tea: Try Fermented Instant Tea from Pique tea. (http://on.bozmd.com/teas) I don't like instant tea, but I like Pique Tea.

OR

2. Drink Ketones-in-a-Can. If you can't seem to reach for the boring drinks yet, or you need a break from boring drinks, swallow ketones. This is a great hack to keep your cells using ketones and advancing your metabolism, while your mind wraps around calorie-free drinks.

CHALLENGE FOR DAY 9:

- Open the can of sardines.

- Mix in mustard, mayonnaise, and onions. Try one bite! The official challenge is to eat the whole can of sardines, but one bite is the first step.

- Post a picture to others. Sardines need some positive advertising. This is one of two foods that I recommend to optimize keto nutrition. Two cans a week is a long-term great goal.

CHALLENGE FOR DAY 10:

Have you found an accountability partner yet? Document when you do. It is worth repeating, accountability partners don't last forever. They are intended for a season. Some seasons are longer than others. Start with a 6-week commitment.

CHALLENGE FOR DAY 11:

- Soak in magnesium: Epsom salt bath or float. In the chart, write down which magnesium float you selected. Document your length of time and the concentration of magnesium.
- Example: 6 cups of Epsom Salt in a 60 min bath

CHALLENGE FOR DAY 12:

Craving versus hunger. You should not be hungry. I want you feeling full thanks to plenty of fat-made hormones.

- Fill out the 10-Minute Food Craving Exercise in Section 2.8 for this challenge.
- Document the date you did the Cravings exercise. Much like tasting sardines, the benefit hides in actually doing the challenge.

CHALLENGE FOR DAY 13:

- Watch the Sleep Lecture by Dr. Boz Find the lecture at this address: http://on.bozmd.com/sleep
- Fill out the Sleep Handout found at this address: http://on.bozmd.com/sleepHO
- Document your total hours of sleep with the chart below. For repeats of Challenge 13, recalculate and document this sleep chart.

Assess your sleep from last night: (Don't cherry-pick your night. Use last night.)

Sleep Awareness Worksheet	
What time did you go to bed last night?	
What time did you wake up?	
How many hours did you sleep last night?	
How many times did you awaken?	
Subtract 1 hour of sleep for each time you woke up.	
Total hours of estimated sleep	

CHALLENGE FOR DAY 14:

Social Success

The impact from COVID-19 changed the norms for social interactions. The setting of this challenge changed from a workplace or a social environment outside the home to one inside your home. Have a family dinner and don't do what you normally do: eat and drink everything. Test yourself. Can you say no to all the food and drinks? Can you deny the food? What happens if you drink salty broth while the family eats?

These social pressures are real! Take the challenge one tiny step at a time. Document your social stress and how you did.

Test your strength. Society resists change—no matter if it's your family or workmates. Your new way of eating creates waves of anxiety in others. How do you respond to their reaction? They are not giving up carbs...you are. Yet, the impact you have on their ecosphere is palpable. Observe their reaction. Document yours. Use the 10-minute Craving Exercise to help capture your experience.

Consider the Cake-Creator that offers, "Just a bite. It won't hurt you."

Or, someone offering you an apple, coaxing you, "Fruit is healthy." She feels the impact of your new choice. Your refusal to accept affects her. This is real. Push your feet into the ground and cram your hands into your pockets to keep from reaching for the forbidden food. Imagine it's poisonous. Throw caution to the wind. Freak her out by grabbing a slab of butter. Eat that right in front of her. Tell her it's your snack. You might be evaluated for sanity—a chunk of butter over an apple. What's wrong with you?

No matter where you conduct this challenge, I love what students learn when they study these situations.

Attract supporters. Don't bristle folks with your new way of eating. **Stay out of the fight.**

Polite phrases to say NO

1. No. I gave up carbs. Please don't tempt me.
2. No. I am allergic to that.
3. No. Gluten might be causing some of my medical problems. I am going without that for a while.
4. No.
5. No. My blood numbers have been high—that's against the rules.

    The number I am thinking about insulin. The fastest way to lower insulin is no food. The second fastest is no carbs.

CHALLENGE FOR DAY 15:

- What is your weight? FIND your BMI. Document your BMI using the chart found in Section 1.3.

- Limit weigh-ins to every other week. Once a month is even better. Stay away from this measuring tool on a daily basis. Measure your weight at the same time of the day.

HEIGHT		WEIGHT																								
		120	130	140	150	160	170	180	190	200	210	220	230	240	250	260	270	280	290	300	310	320	330	340	360	380	400
5'0"	23	25	27	29	31	33	35	37	39	41	43	45	47	49	51	53	55	57	59	61	63	65	66	70	74	78
5'1"	23	25	27	28	30	32	34	36	38	40	42	44	45	47	49	51	53	55	57	59	61	62	64	68	71	75
5'2"	22	24	26	27	29	31	33	35	37	38	40	42	44	46	48	49	51	53	55	57	59	60	62	65	69	73
5'3"	21	23	25	27	28	30	32	34	36	37	39	41	43	44	46	48	50	51	53	55	57	59	60	63	67	70
5'4"	21	22	24	26	28	29	31	33	34	36	38	40	41	43	45	46	48	50	52	53	55	57	58	61	65	68
5'5"	20	22	23	25	27	28	30	32	33	35	37	38	40	42	43	45	47	48	50	52	53	55	56	60	63	67
5'6"	19	21	23	24	26	27	29	31	32	34	36	37	39	40	42	44	45	47	49	50	52	53	55	58	61	64
5'7"	19	20	22	24	25	27	28	30	31	33	35	36	38	39	41	42	44	46	47	49	50	52	53	56	60	63
5'8"	18	20	21	23	24	26	27	29	30	32	34	35	37	38	40	41	43	44	46	47	49	50	52	55	58	61
5'9"	18	19	21	22	24	25	27	28	30	31	33	34	36	37	38	40	41	43	44	46	47	49	50	53	56	59
5'10"	17	19	20	22	23	24	26	27	29	30	32	33	35	36	37	39	40	42	43	45	46	47	49	52	55	57
5'11"	17	18	20	21	22	24	25	27	28	29	31	32	34	35	36	38	39	41	42	43	45	46	47	50	53	56
6'0"	16	18	19	20	22	23	24	26	27	29	30	31	33	34	35	37	38	39	41	42	43	45	46	49	52	54
6'1"	16	17	19	20	21	22	24	25	26	28	29	30	32	33	34	36	37	38	40	41	42	44	45	48	50	53
6'2"	15	17	18	19	21	22	23	24	26	27	28	30	31	32	33	35	36	37	39	40	41	42	44	46	49	51
6'3"	15	16	18	19	20	21	23	24	25	26	28	29	30	31	33	34	35	36	38	39	40	41	43	45	48	50
6'4"	15	16	17	18	20	21	22	23	24	26	27	28	29	30	32	33	34	35	37	38	39	40	41	44	46	49
6'5"	14	15	17	18	19	20	21	23	24	25	26	27	29	30	31	32	33	34	36	37	38	39	40	43	45	47
6'6"	14	15	16	17	19	20	21	22	23	24	25	27	28	29	30	31	32	34	35	36	37	38	39	42	44	46
6'7"	14	15	16	17	18	19	20	21	23	24	25	26	27	28	29	30	32	33	34	35	36	37	38	41	43	45
6'8"	13	14	15	17	18	19	20	21	22	23	24	25	26	28	29	30	31	32	33	34	35	36	37	39	42	44
6'9"	13	14	15	16	17	18	19	20	21	23	24	25	26	27	28	29	30	31	32	33	34	35	36	39	41	43
6'10"	13	14	15	16	17	18	19	20	21	22	23	24	25	26	27	28	29	30	31	32	34	35	35	38	40	42

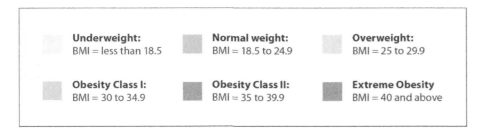

Underweight: BMI = less than 18.5	**Normal weight:** BMI = 18.5 to 24.9	**Overweight:** BMI = 25 to 29.9
Obesity Class I: BMI = 30 to 34.9	**Obesity Class II:** BMI = 35 to 39.9	**Extreme Obesity** BMI = 40 and above

Fill out this chart on your second week.

Date	Time	Blood Pressure	Heart Rate	PeeTone Strip Color	Total Carbs	Bowel Activity	Challenge Completed
				0 1 2 3 4 5 6			
				0 1 2 3 4 5 6			
				0 1 2 3 4 5 6			
				0 1 2 3 4 5 6			
				0 1 2 3 4 5 6			
				0 1 2 3 4 5 6			
				0 1 2 3 4 5 6			
				0 1 2 3 4 5 6			
				0 1 2 3 4 5 6			
				0 1 2 3 4 5 6			
				0 1 2 3 4 5 6			
				0 1 2 3 4 5 6			
				0 1 2 3 4 5 6			
				0 1 2 3 4 5 6			
				0 1 2 3 4 5 6			

ketoCONTINUUM Workbook

Fill out this chart on your second week the second time around.

Date	Time	Blood Pressure	Heart Rate	PeeTone Strip Color	Total Carbs	Bowel Activity	Challenge Completed
				0 1 2 3 4 5 6			
				0 1 2 3 4 5 6			
				0 1 2 3 4 5 6			
				0 1 2 3 4 5 6			
				0 1 2 3 4 5 6			
				0 1 2 3 4 5 6			
				0 1 2 3 4 5 6			
				0 1 2 3 4 5 6			
				0 1 2 3 4 5 6			
				0 1 2 3 4 5 6			
				0 1 2 3 4 5 6			
				0 1 2 3 4 5 6			
				0 1 2 3 4 5 6			
				0 1 2 3 4 5 6			
				0 1 2 3 4 5 6			
				0 1 2 3 4 5 6			

3.2 KETO**CONTINUUM #3**

ketoCONTINUUM	GUIDELINES	NEXT STEPS
#3: I "accidentally" missed a meal. [Keto-adapted]	Fat supplies the resources needed to make fat-built hormones approach healthy levels. Appetite decreases according to body's chemistry.	Sometimes it takes 10 weeks before this moment happens. Don't look at the scale. Listen for absence of hunger.

BEGINNERS: KETO**CONTINUUM**S #1–#4

Eat less than 20 grams of total carbs per day.
This, in addition to eating high fat, shifts your chemistry to a ketogenic state. Ketone chemistry will carry you the first part of this process.
Pee ketones. Reduce the frequency with which you check ketones. Just ensure that you are making them. As long as ketones remain present, your chemistry will carry you through ketoCONTINUUM #3.

Once you accidentally miss a meal, find the right timing to do the following:

1) Advance to ketoCONTINUUM #4
2) Add gentle exercise. Start with a walk. Slowly progress in the intensity and frequency.
   Consider setting a goal of sweating for 15 minutes three times a week.

Baseline Metabolism:
Rarely happens by week 3-4

Stressing Metabolism:
Don't stress your metabolism yet.

	ketoCONTINUUM	WHO DOES THE WORK?	TEST
BEGINNER	**#1:** I eat every 2–4 hours	CHEMISTRY CARRIES YOU	X
	#2: LESS THAN 20 total carbs		Urine PeeTone Strips
	#3: I "accidentally" missed a meal. [Keto-adapted]		
BASELINE METABOLISM	**#4:** Eat 2 meals per day	YOU DO THE WORK. Discipline needed for each new step.	
	#5: 16:8		
	#6: Advanced 16:8		
	#7: 23:1 OMAD ALL in one hour		
	#8: Advanced 23:1/OMAD		
STRESSING METABOLISM	**#9:** 36-hour fast	PSYCHOLOGY. Use tribe for best results.	Blood Ketone Strips
	#10: 36-hour fast without a celebration meal		
	#11: 48-hour fast		
	#12: 72-hour fast		

Fill this chart on your third week. Watch for the moment you "accidentally miss a meal.'"

WEEK 3	Day 1	Day 2	Day 3	Day 4	Day 5	Day 6	Day 7
Blood Pressure							
PeeTones							
Symptoms of Low Magnesium							
Epsom Salt Bath/Float							
Accountability Partner Check-in							
Number of Unsweetened Drinks							
Meal 1 Time							
Meal 2 Time							
Meal 3 Time							
I accidentally missed a meal							
Hours Slept							
Weight (Only once/ week)							

WEEK 4	Day 1	Day 2	Day 3	Day 4	Day 5	Day 6	Day 7
Blood Pressure							
PeeTones							
Symptoms of Low Magnesium							
Epsom Salt Bath/Float							
Accountability Partner Check-in							
Number of Unsweetened Drinks							
Meal 1 Time							
Meal 2 Time							
Meal 3 Time							
I accidentally missed a meal							
Hours Slept							
Weight (Only once/ week)							

WEEK 5	Day 1	Day 2	Day 3	Day 4	Day 5	Day 6	Day 7
Blood Pressure							
PeeTones							
Symptoms of Low Magnesium							
Epsom Salt Bath/Float							
Accountability Partner Check-in							
Number of Unsweetened Drinks							
Meal 1 Time							
Meal 2 Time							
Meal 3 Time							
I accidentally missed a meal							
Hours Slept							
Weight (Only once/ week)							

3.3 KETOCONTINUUM #4

ketoCONTINUUM	GUIDELINES	NEXT STEPS
#4: Eat 2 meals per day	Choose to eat only 2 meals per day.	Succeed 7 days in a row before advancing.

BEWARE:

Some find ketoCONTINUUM #4 a challenge to their identity. Years of cleaned plates and scheduled meals shaped their thoughts about meals.

They never missed a meal. N.E.V.E.R. One participant continued to eat three square meals a day even though he bragged about no hunger. Another person in the keto-support group drew praise and cheers when she skipped her first meal. Only then did he consider following her example.

Use these tips when mastering ketoCONTINUUM #4:

- Eating only two meals a day is a choice. Plan your two mealtimes.

- Replace your missing mealtime with a SUBSTITUTION. Examples: a walk, a card game, a time to journal, or other forms of self-care.

- Skip the meal when you feel the least amount of hunger. This rule changes as you advance along the continuum, but begin with the easiest meal.

- Keep checking your PeeTones. Once a day is enough.

- Eat two meals daily for seven consecutive days before advancing. One day of two daily meals is not a habit.

- Pass the Social stress test in Challenge Day 14 (Section 3.1)

	ketoCONTINUUM	WHO DOES THE WORK?	TEST
BEGINNER	#1: I eat every 2–4 hours	CHEMISTRY CARRIES YOU	X
BEGINNER	#2: LESS THAN 20 total carbs	CHEMISTRY CARRIES YOU	Urine PeeTone Strips
BEGINNER	#3: I "accidentally" missed a meal. [Keto-adapted]	CHEMISTRY CARRIES YOU	Urine PeeTone Strips
BASELINE METABOLISM	#4: Eat 2 meals per day	YOU DO THE WORK. Discipline needed for each new step.	Urine PeeTone Strips
BASELINE METABOLISM	#5: 16:8	YOU DO THE WORK. Discipline needed for each new step.	Urine PeeTone Strips
BASELINE METABOLISM	#6: Advanced 16:8	YOU DO THE WORK. Discipline needed for each new step.	Urine PeeTone Strips
BASELINE METABOLISM	#7: 23:1 OMAD ALL in one hour	YOU DO THE WORK. Discipline needed for each new step.	Urine PeeTone Strips
BASELINE METABOLISM	#8: Advanced 23:1/OMAD	YOU DO THE WORK. Discipline needed for each new step.	Blood Ketone Strips
STRESSING METABOLISM	#9: 36-hour fast	PSYCHOLOGY. Use tribe for best results.	Blood Ketone Strips
STRESSING METABOLISM	#10: 36-hour fast without a celebration meal	PSYCHOLOGY. Use tribe for best results.	Blood Ketone Strips
STRESSING METABOLISM	#11: 48-hour fast	PSYCHOLOGY. Use tribe for best results.	Blood Ketone Strips
STRESSING METABOLISM	#12: 72-hour fast	PSYCHOLOGY. Use tribe for best results.	Blood Ketone Strips

WEEK 6	Day 1	Day 2	Day 3	Day 4	Day 5	Day 6	Day 7
Blood Pressure							
PeeTones							
Symptoms of Low Magnesium							
Epsom Salt Bath/Float							
Accountability Partner Check-in							
Number of Unsweetened Drinks							
Meal 1 Time							
Meal 2 Time							
Consecutive Days of 2 Meals Per Day	1 2 3 4 5 6 7	1 2 3 4 5 6 7	1 2 3 4 5 6 7	1 2 3 4 5 6 7	1 2 3 4 5 6 7	1 2 3 4 5 6 7	1 2 3 4 5 6 7
Hours Slept							
Exercise							
Weight (Only once/ week)							

WEEK 7	Day 1	Day 2	Day 3	Day 4	Day 5	Day 6	Day 7
Blood Pressure							
PeeTones							
Symptoms of Low Magnesium							
Epsom Salt Bath/Float							
Accountability Partner Check-in							
Number of Unsweetened Drinks							
Meal 1 Time							
Meal 2 Time							
Consecutive Days of 2 Meals Per Day	1 2 3 4 5 6 7	1 2 3 4 5 6 7	1 2 3 4 5 6 7	1 2 3 4 5 6 7	1 2 3 4 5 6 7	1 2 3 4 5 6 7	1 2 3 4 5 6 7
Hours Slept							
Exercise							
Weight (Only once/ week)							

WEEK 8	Day 1	Day 2	Day 3	Day 4	Day 5	Day 6	Day 7
Blood Pressure							
PeeTones							
Symptoms of Low Magnesium							
Epsom Salt Bath/Float							
Accountability Partner Check-in							
Number of Unsweetened Drinks							
Meal 1 Time							
Meal 2 Time							
Consecutive Days of 2 Meals Per Day	1 2 3 4 5 6 7	1 2 3 4 5 6 7	1 2 3 4 5 6 7	1 2 3 4 5 6 7	1 2 3 4 5 6 7	1 2 3 4 5 6 7	1 2 3 4 5 6 7
Hours Slept							
Exercise							
Weight (Only once/ week)							

ketoCONTINUUM

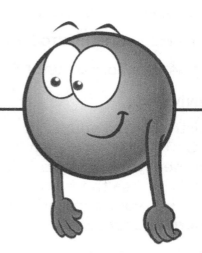

SECTION

4

BASELINE METABOLISM

4.1   Overview of Baseline Metabolisms

4.2   ketoCONTINUUM #5

4.3   Measuring Ketones & Dr. Boz Ratio

4.4   ketoCONTINUUM #6

4.5   ketoCONTINUUM #7

4.6   ketoCONTINUUM #8

BozMD.com

4.1 OVERVIEW OF BASELINE METABOLISMS

BEGINNERS: KETOCONTINUUMS #1–#4

BASELINE METABOLISM: KETOCONTINUUMS #5–#8

STRESSING METABOLISM: KETOCONTINUUMS #9–#12

BEGINNERS:

Chemistry carried you.
ketoCONTINUUM #1-4 shifted your chemistry. You replenished your storage tank of fat-built hormones. Your cellular health begins to improve. During these 4 continuums, your crippled mitochondria improved and your hormones rose.

BASELINE METABOLISMS:

Metabolism stands for the exercise your cells get at a microscopic level. Metabolic health measures the strength of your cells to function. Metabolic health measures how well your cells do at life.

Think of ketoCONTINUUM #5-8 as the general exercise needed for your mitochondria. These continuums step through a progression that slowly builds metabolism. Energy production within your cells improves on each of these continuums — you make more energy and can respond rapidly to changing demands. These baseline options deliver enough energy to meet life's needs such as infections, broken bones, reversal of fatigue, and reducing inflammation. If you never advance beyond these 4 stages, your life would be mostly healthy.

	ketoCONTINUUM	WHO DOES THE WORK?	TEST
BEGINNER	**#1:** I eat every 2–4 hours	CHEMISTRY CARRIES YOU	X
	#2: LESS THAN 20 total carbs		Urine PeeTone Strips
	#3: I "accidentally" missed a meal. [Keto-adapted]		
	#4: Eat 2 meals per day	YOU DO THE WORK. Discipline needed for each new step.	
BASELINE METABOLISM	**#5:** 16:8		
	#6: Advanced 16:8		
	#7: 23:1 OMAD ALL in one hour		
	#8: Advanced 23:1/OMAD	PSYCHOLOGY. Use tribe for best results.	Blood Ketone Strips
STRESSING METABOLISM	**#9:** 36-hour fast		
	#10: 36-hour fast without a celebration meal		
	#11: 48-hour fast		
	#12: 72-hour fast		

ketoCONTINUUMs #5–8 reflect eating patterns linked to longevity and restored health. Your baseline metabolism for longevity should be one of these 4.

When patients arrive with years of broken health, I encourage them to find one of these baselines that fit into their current season. Stay at that baseline. Period. Stay there.

ketoCONTINUUM #5

16:8 Eat ALL food in an 8-hour window.

- Eat ALL food, snacks, and supplements in an 8-hour window. No eating, snacking or chewing for 16 hours.

- That means no gum during fasting hours. Suck on salt if you need a substitute. Keep your coffee filled with fat.

ketoCONTINUUM #6

Advanced 16:8 Conquered morning drink [calorie-free and sweetener-free]

- Clean up your morning drink. Remove all calories and sweeteners.
  Morning drink = no fat, no MCT, no butter, no sweeteners, no calories.
  16 hours = only salt, water, black coffee, or tea.

- Don't remove the fat from your morning drink before this phase. You needed it to get here. Once you get here, it's time to let it go.

ketoCONTINUUM #7

23:1 OMAD: One Meal A Day. ALL CALORIES IN ONE hour. 23 hours = none.

- ALL calories and sweeteners in one hour.
  23 hours = Only salt, water, tea, or coffee.

- Begin checking blood numbers right before you eat.

ketoCONTINUUM #8:

- Advanced 23:1/OMAD...Move eating hour within 11 hours of sunrise.

- Move you eating-hour within 11 hours following sunrise to match your circadian rhythm.

Record your Dr. Boz Ratio first thing in the morning. Repeat before eating.

Restoring health at an electron level takes time. It can take a couple of years to advance through these four continuums.

The timeline depends on your skills. Skills for saying no. Skills for addressing social settings peppered with temptations. Skills for getting enough sleep at night. It's not a race. These metabolic stages should be practiced. Together, we will slowly improve those skills to strengthen your mitochondria. The support around you becomes critical during times of change. Support groups matter.

WHAT SEASON OF LIFE ARE YOU IN?

Life has seasons. If this is the season where your daughter is getting married and you want to rush to remove weight, STOP. Sprinting through ketoCONTINUUM stages proves ill-advised. The improvement to metabolic health happens steadily. How stable is this season of your life?

Read this list of the most stressful times of life. How many do you identify with during this season of your life? Tread slowly. This is not a race. The turtle wins.

- Divorce/Marital separation
- Imprisonment
- Trouble with the law
- Death of a close family member
- Personal injury or illness
- Wedding
- Marital reconciliation
- Moving
- Job loss/Career change
- Initiation of retirement

- Change in health of family member
- Pregnancy
- Sex difficulties
- Son or daughter leaving home
- Gain of a new family member
- Business adjustments
- Change in financial state
- Trouble with in-laws
- Death of a close friend

Mastery of BASELINE METABOLISM takes discipline, metabolic understanding, and support. Each one takes education and self-reflection. As you progress through ketoCONTINUUMs #5–8, your metabolism strengthens. By ketoCONTINUUM #8 you will tap into some advanced psychology.

Do not underestimate these steps. These advancements break a weight-loss stall, repair immunity, and spark autophagy. They deliver on that promise when keto-chemistry is stable and persistent.

SUPPORT GROUPS

Support equals success. Joining a keto support group makes you stronger together. Support groups usually sound like something someone else needs. Support groups are not filled with perfect partners. They are filled with others who try. You are stronger together.

ANALYZE YOUR REASONS FOR EATING.

The first few days you ate less than 20 total carbs, you lowered your insulin and induced many chemistry changes. By days three, four, and five, the change in chemistry slowed down, but the reality of remaining low-carb had not settled into your brain. What seemed novel on those first days of keto quickly evolved into a personal battle inside your mind

Use the Craving Analysis Exercise in Section 2.8 to study yourself.

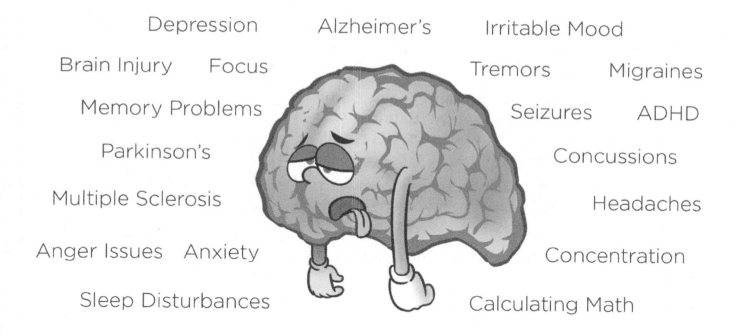

4.2 KETO**CONTINUUM** #5

ketoCONTINUUM	GUIDELINES	NEXT STEPS
#5: 16:8	Eat ALL food, snacks and supplements in an 8-hour window. No eating, snacking or chewing for 16 hours.	That means no gum during fasting hours. Suck on salt if you need a substitute. Keep your coffee filled with fat.

16 + 8 = 24   16:8

WHY DOESN'T THE FAT COME FROM THE FAT CELLS?

Fat cells follow the command of insulin. Insulin instructs when to open and close the gates of fat cells. Only when the gates open will your body use fats as fuel.

The first 4 ketoCONTINUUMs added fat through your mouth. Fat came in, carbs stopped entering and your insulin production decreased.

Low carb intake dropped your insulin initially. Some fat cells released their stored energy. Eating twice daily dropped insulin further. Another crop of fat cells opened their doors of storage.

Each time your abundant insulin notches downward, your chemistry changes. Each improvement opens more fat fuel.

- Advance your chemistry to tap into your next layer of storage.

- Ratchet your chemistry to 16:8.

- Sixteen hours of your day without food.

- Eight hours where you can eat.

- Eight hours you sleep. Limit all eating to 8 consecutive hours. That means beyond the hours you spend sleeping, you need 8 hours when you DON'T eat.

	ketoCONTINUUM	WHO DOES THE WORK?	TEST
BEGINNER	**#1:** I eat every 2–4 hours	CHEMISTRY CARRIES YOU	X
	#2: LESS THAN 20 total carbs		Urine PeeTone Strips
	#3: I "accidentally" missed a meal. [Keto-adapted]		
	#4: Eat 2 meals per day	YOU DO THE WORK. Discipline needed for each new step.	
BASELINE METABOLISM	**#5:** 16:8		
	#6: Advanced 16:8		
	#7: 23:1 OMAD ALL in one hour		
	#8: Advanced 23:1/OMAD		
STRESSING METABOLISM	**#9:** 36-hour fast	PSYCHOLOGY. Use tribe for best results.	Blood Ketone Strips
	#10: 36-hour fast without a celebration meal		
	#11: 48-hour fast		
	#12: 72-hour fast		

The block of time when you eat starts at one time and then stops eight hours later. From sunrise to sunset, you can't start and stop the eating clock. Put your fasting hours on either side of your eating window. Once keto-adapted, restrict the hours you eat. This advances you to the next layer of chemistry. Food enters your body only during those eight hours. Then stop. This requires a conscious choice. Make this decision when you are ready. Choose the next step.

HOW LONG?

Stay at ketoCONTINUUM #5 until you master it. Mastery centers around the removal of cravings. You will know you are good when your brain stops asking for food outside of those eight hours.

You will not wake up tomorrow armed with the skills to conquer all these challenges. You are likely not aware of the challenges until they punch you in the nose. Temptation sneaks up on you.

Celebrate seven consecutive days before even considering ketoCONTINUUM #6. Use the chart on the next page to keep track of the time spent eating versus fasting. The chart for ketoCONTINUUM #5 offers a generous eating window of 16 hours. Use the graph in the middle column to shade in the hours you eat.

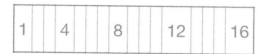

If you kept your eating within eight hours, do a little dance. Then circle the YES. Use the next column to help you track how many days in a row you limited your eating to eight hours.

Notice that no column for PeeTones strips is in this chart. Also notice that I have not asked you to start checking blood numbers yet. This is purposeful. Although keto chemistry remains important, mastering this skill is even more important. Without the ability to refrain from eating for 16 consecutive hours, you will plateau your healing.

The ketoCONTINUUM #5 skill takes time to master - especially if you've been addicted to food. Be gentle with yourself if you struggle. Remind yourself that you are learning a new skill. If you can't seem to break the habit of eating within eight hours, use the 10-Minute-Craving Exercise from Section 2.8.

Jot down the time the moment you first CHEW something. Stop chewing or swallowing all food 8 hours after the first bite. Drinks don't count during this phase, but I encourage you to keep track of them. If you have drinks with calories or sweeteners in them, add a tally mark to the right column.

Before fasting or advancing to ketoCONTINUUM #6, succeed at ketoCONTINUUM #5 for 7 consecutive days.

Date	TIME: First Bite	TIME: Last Bite	Did you keep the food within 8 hours?	How many days in a row did you keep to 8 hours of consumption?	# of drinks with calories or sweeteners
			Yes/No 1 4 8 12 16	1 2 3 4 5 6 7	
			Yes/No 1 4 8 12 16	1 2 3 4 5 6 7	
			Yes/No 1 4 8 12 16	1 2 3 4 5 6 7	
			Yes/No 1 4 8 12 16	1 2 3 4 5 6 7	
			Yes/No 1 4 8 12 16	1 2 3 4 5 6 7	
			Yes/No 1 4 8 12 16	1 2 3 4 5 6 7	
			Yes/No 1 4 8 12 16	1 2 3 4 5 6 7	
			Yes/No 1 4 8 12 16	1 2 3 4 5 6 7	
			Yes/No 1 4 8 12 16	1 2 3 4 5 6 7	

ketoCONTINUUM Workbook

ketoCONTINUUM #5

Date	TIME: First Bite	TIME: Last Bite	Did you keep the food within 8 hours?	How many days in a row did you keep to 8 hours of consumption?	# of drinks with calories or sweeteners
			Yes/No 1 4 8 12 16	1 2 3 4 5 6 7	
			Yes/No 1 4 8 12 16	1 2 3 4 5 6 7	
			Yes/No 1 4 8 12 16	1 2 3 4 5 6 7	
			Yes/No 1 4 8 12 16	1 2 3 4 5 6 7	
			Yes/No 1 4 8 12 16	1 2 3 4 5 6 7	
			Yes/No 1 4 8 12 16	1 2 3 4 5 6 7	
			Yes/No 1 4 8 12 16	1 2 3 4 5 6 7	
			Yes/No 1 4 8 12 16	1 2 3 4 5 6 7	
			Yes/No 1 4 8 12 16	1 2 3 4 5 6 7	
			Yes/No 1 4 8 12 16	1 2 3 4 5 6 7	
			Yes/No 1 4 8 12 16	1 2 3 4 5 6 7	

ketoCONTINUUM #5

Date	TIME: First Bite	TIME: Last Bite	Did you keep the food within 8 hours?	How many days in a row did you keep to 8 hours of consumption?	# of drinks with calories or sweeteners
			Yes/No 1 4 8 12 16	1 2 3 4 5 6 7	
			Yes/No 1 4 8 12 16	1 2 3 4 5 6 7	
			Yes/No 1 4 8 12 16	1 2 3 4 5 6 7	
			Yes/No 1 4 8 12 16	1 2 3 4 5 6 7	
			Yes/No 1 4 8 12 16	1 2 3 4 5 6 7	
			Yes/No 1 4 8 12 16	1 2 3 4 5 6 7	
			Yes/No 1 4 8 12 16	1 2 3 4 5 6 7	
			Yes/No 1 4 8 12 16	1 2 3 4 5 6 7	
			Yes/No 1 4 8 12 16	1 2 3 4 5 6 7	
			Yes/No 1 4 8 12 16	1 2 3 4 5 6 7	
			Yes/No 1 4 8 12 16	1 2 3 4 5 6 7	

ketoCONTINUUM #5

Date	TIME: First Bite	TIME: Last Bite	Did you keep the food within 8 hours?	How many days in a row did you keep to 8 hours of consumption?	# of drinks with calories or sweeteners
			Yes/No 1 4 8 12 16	1 2 3 4 5 6 7	
			Yes/No 1 4 8 12 16	1 2 3 4 5 6 7	
			Yes/No 1 4 8 12 16	1 2 3 4 5 6 7	
			Yes/No 1 4 8 12 16	1 2 3 4 5 6 7	
			Yes/No 1 4 8 12 16	1 2 3 4 5 6 7	
			Yes/No 1 4 8 12 16	1 2 3 4 5 6 7	
			Yes/No 1 4 8 12 16	1 2 3 4 5 6 7	
			Yes/No 1 4 8 12 16	1 2 3 4 5 6 7	
			Yes/No 1 4 8 12 16	1 2 3 4 5 6 7	
			Yes/No 1 4 8 12 16	1 2 3 4 5 6 7	
			Yes/No 1 4 8 12 16	1 2 3 4 5 6 7	

4.3 Measuring Ketones & Dr Boz Ratio

Transition from urine PeeTone strips to measuring blood ketones.
Read through this chart.

	HOW TO TEST YOUR KETONES		
Type of Test	URINE TESTING	BREATH TESTING	BLOOD TESTING
Pros	Best for beginners Least expensive Results in seconds	Easy to use if you have healthy lungs Pretty good accuracy One-time cost	Extremely accurate Direct measurements of ketones as a fuel
Cons	Measures extra ketones being used as fuel Negative results can be an error	Not good for patients with asthma or weak lungs Measures extra ketones, not ketones being used as fuel	Most expensive Requires a finger prick —not for the faint of heart
Highlights	Best for beginners. Use this to prove you're in ketosis. Not as accurate at reflecting how much you're in ketosis	Breath testing is more accurate than urine testing, but less accurate than blood testing. The biggest plus is you don't have to keep buying lancets or strips—buy it once and you're set.	The absolute most accurate result. Use this once you've been keto-adapted as a real-time and accurate way to keep yourself accountable or after a long fast to get your Dr. Boz Ratio.
The Verdict	Beginners should use urine test strips. After you're keto-adapted, start using a blood test to get real-time and accurate results. This also allows you to calculate your Dr. Boz Ratio.		

It's time to advance to blood testing of ketones and glucose. Invest in a meter that allows home testing of these two biomarkers. Several meters on the market allow you to test both metrics with one meter. Glucose test strips measure the glucose in circulation and ketone test strips measure the beta hydroxybutyrate. These strips are sold separately. I recommend the brand ForaCare because of their uniquely stable test strips. I have personally tossed out other brands of test strips that defected when accidentally left in a freezing or overheated car.

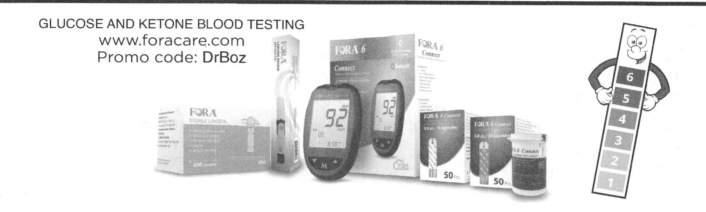

GLUCOSE AND KETONE BLOOD TESTING
www.foracare.com
Promo code: DrBoz

DR. BOZ RATIO

The Dr. Boz Ratio (DBR) is a calculation from the biomarkers blood glucose and blood ketones. This metric tracks your metabolic health. Read the full explanation in Chapter 24 of ketoCONTINUUM. (Notice the header on this page that correlates to the book's chapter.) Take notice in the graph below that the metrics for glucose and ketones do not match. The DBR was derived from the Glucose Ketone Index (GKI) which uses both ketone and glucose measurements in mmol/L. Since glucose is measured in mg/dL in the United States, the DBR simplifies the calculation without converting the units of glucose from mg/dL to mmol/L.

Dividing your blood glucose by your blood ketones approximates your metabolism and insulin resistance. The lower your DBR, the lower your insulin resistance, and the healthier your mitochondria. Due to the natural variability in these blood biomarkers, the ratio of the paired numbers offers a clearer understanding of what's happening inside your body.

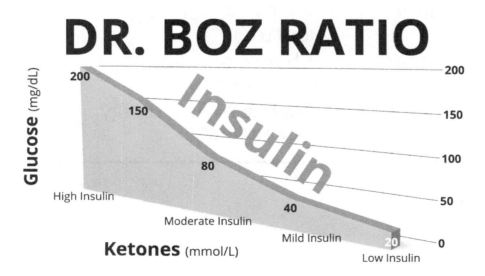

DBR GOALS

The best time to measure DBR is first thing in the morning or right before breaking a fast. Another useful time to measure your DBR is about 90 minutes after stressing your mitochondria from exercise or sauna.

DBR measurements taken during those times can predict the strength of your metabolism. A DBR of 80 suggests a weight loss zone. If you are using keto-chemistry to open your fat cells and lose weight, set your DBR goal to 80 or less.

A DBR of 40 boasts of a stronger army of mitochondria. This ratio reflects the power to repair from chronic issues like a sluggish immune system or autoimmune disorders such as psoriasis or inflammatory bowel diseases.

The highest achievement is a DBR of 20 or less. When metabolisms reach this level of performance, amazing results unfold. This target resolves extreme health issues where advanced levels of autophagy are needed. Many cancer patients live here during the most intense seasons of their recovery. Several patients reversing severe brain disorders use this advanced level to enhance the repair of their brain. Please do not do this without the close supervision of a physician.

DR. BOZ RATIO
Glucose ÷ Ketones

Under 80: Might Get Autophagy
WEIGHT LOSS
Under 40: Solid Chance of Autophagy
REPAIR OF IMMUNE SYSTEM
Under 20: Best Chance of Autophagy
GOAL FOR CANCER PATIENTS

DBR COMPARED TO GKI

The chart below shows the flow of data to calculate the Glucose:Ketone Index (GKI) and the Dr. Boz Ratio (DBR.) Under the glucose column, glucose is documented using both metrics: mg/dl and the mmol/L. Ketones are measured in mmol/L.

GKI: The Glucose Ketone Index provides the ratio of glucose to ketones using mmol/L for both biomarkers. Glucose divided by ketones yields the amount of glucose per mmol/L of ketones. In order to compare one GKI to the next, the ketones are converted to a common denominator of 1.0 mmol/L .This results in a Glucose:Ketone ratio of X:1. Commonly the ketone number is dropped off because it is always reported as 1.0. The remaining glucose metric is reported as the GKI. Example from the first row = GKI of 4.4.

DBR: The Dr. Boz Ratio is calculated with the numeric value of glucose using mg/dl divided by the ketones in mmol/L.

Glucose	Ketones	Dr. Boz Ratio	GKI	Zone
96 mg/dL 5.3 mmol/L	1.2	80	5.3 : 1.2 **4.4 : 1**	Weight Loss
99 mg/dL 5.5 mmol/L	1.5	66	5.5 : 1.5 **3.7 : 1**	Weight Loss
75 mg/dL 4.2 mmol/L	0.9	83	4.2 : 0.9 **4.7 : 1**	Nearly Weight Loss
88 mg/dL 4.9 mmol/L	1.1	80	4.9 : 1.1 **4.5 : 1**	Weight Loss
76 mg/dL 4.2 mmol/L	2.1	36	4.2 : 2.1 **2.0 : 1**	Immune Repair
60 mg/dL 3.3 mmol/L	3.0	20	3.3 : 3.2 **1.0 : 1**	Critical Care

CLASSIC DR.BOZ CHART: Use this chart to practice calculating your Dr. Boz Ratio.

Date:	Time of Measurement	# Hours Fasting	Glucose mg/dL	Glucose mmol/L	Ketone mmol/L	Glucose:Ketone Index	Dr. Boz Ratio	Minutes of Exercise/Sauna	Blood Pressure

David, from the story in *ketoCONTINUUM*, tracked his progress using this chart.

Heart Rate	Weight (limit to weekly)	Total Hours Slept	Total Carbs Protein Grams	Meal Time(s) / Notes

Date:	Time of Measurement	# Hours Fasting	Glucose mg/dL	Glucose mmol/L	Ketone mmol/L	Glucose:Ketone Index	Dr. Boz Ratio	Minutes of Exercise/Sauna	Blood Pressure

ketoCONTINUUM Workbook

Heart Rate	Weight (limit to weekly)	Total Hours Slept	Total Carbs Protein Grams	Meal Time(s) / Notes

Date:	Time of Measurement	# Hours Fasting	Glucose mg/dL	Glucose mmol/L	Ketone mmol/L	Glucose:Ketone Index	Dr. Boz Ratio	Minutes of Exercise/Sauna	Blood Pressure

ketoCONTINUUM Workbook

Heart Rate	Weight (limit to weekly)	Total Hours Slept	Total Carbs Protein Grams	Meal Time(s) / Notes

Date:	Time of Measurement	# Hours Fasting	Glucose mg/dL	Glucose mmol/L	Ketone mmol/L	Glucose:Ketone Index	Dr. Boz Ratio	Minutes of Exercise/Sauna	Blood Pressure

ketoCONTINUUM Workbook

Heart Rate	Weight (limit to weekly)	Total Hours Slept	Total Carbs Protein Grams	Meal Time(s) / Notes

4.4 KETOCONTINUUM #6

ketoCONTINUUM	GUIDELINES	NEXT STEPS
#6: Advanced 16:8	Clean up your morning drink. Remove all calories and sweeteners. Morning drink = no fat, no MCT, no butter, no sweeteners, no calories. The 16 hours = only salt, water, black coffee or tea.	Don't remove the fat from your morning drink before this phase. You needed it to get here. Now it's time to let it go.

It is time to address those lovely morning fat-filled drinks.

ketoCONTINUUM #6 continues the practice of limiting consumption to eight hours per day as practiced in #5. Clean up your morning drink.
TRANSLATION: Remove all calories and sweeteners from your morning drink. That means no fat, no MCT, no butter, no sweeteners, no calories.

16 hours = salt, water, black coffee, or tea.

If you're not ready to surrender those delicious drinks in the morning, there is another option. If you keep your keto coffee, start your eight-hour timer when you first sip of that drink.

The chart for ketoCONTINUUM #6 facilitates restricted-calorie consumption to 8 hours. Set the timer for 8 hours when you consume the first calorie. Use a timer to respect this firm boundary. When the timer rings, all food consumption stops.

Documenting seven consecutive successful days correlates to the greatest success for advanced stressors of your metabolism.

Notice the absence of a column for ketones. Feel free to monitor your ketones or your Dr. Boz Ratio. This section focuses on conquering the skill of time-restricted eating. Master this skill before advancing. There will be plenty of time to follow your DBR once you've mastered this.

	ketoCONTINUUM	WHO DOES THE WORK?	TEST
BEGINNER	**#1:** I eat every 2–4 hours	CHEMISTRY CARRIES YOU	X
	#2: LESS THAN 20 total carbs		Urine PeeTone Strips
	#3: I "accidentally" missed a meal. [Keto-adapted]		
BASELINE METABOLISM	**#4:** Eat 2 meals per day	YOU DO THE WORK. Discipline needed for each new step.	
	#5: 16:8		
	#6: Advanced 16:8		
	#7: 23:1 OMAD ALL in one hour		
	#8: Advanced 23:1/OMAD		
STRESSING METABOLISM	**#9:** 36-hour fast	PSYCHOLOGY. Use tribe for best results.	Blood Ketone Strips
	#10: 36-hour fast without a celebration meal		
	#11: 48-hour fast		
	#12: 72-hour fast		

Date	TIME: First Bite or Sip (first calorie or sweeteners)		When you will stop all calories, chewing and sweeteners	How many days in a row did you make it?
		Add 8 hours >		1 2 3 4 5 6 7
		Add 8 hours >		1 2 3 4 5 6 7
		Add 8 hours >		1 2 3 4 5 6 7
		Add 8 hours >		1 2 3 4 5 6 7
		Add 8 hours >		1 2 3 4 5 6 7
		Add 8 hours >		1 2 3 4 5 6 7
		Add 8 hours >		1 2 3 4 5 6 7
		Add 8 hours >		1 2 3 4 5 6 7
		Add 8 hours >		1 2 3 4 5 6 7
		Add 8 hours >		1 2 3 4 5 6 7
		Add 8 hours >		1 2 3 4 5 6 7

Date	TIME: First Bite or Sip (first calorie or sweeteners)		When you will stop all calories, chewing and sweeteners	How many days in a row did you make it?
		Add 8 hours >		1 2 3 4 5 6 7
		Add 8 hours >		1 2 3 4 5 6 7
		Add 8 hours >		1 2 3 4 5 6 7
		Add 8 hours >		1 2 3 4 5 6 7
		Add 8 hours >		1 2 3 4 5 6 7
		Add 8 hours >		1 2 3 4 5 6 7
		Add 8 hours >		1 2 3 4 5 6 7
		Add 8 hours >		1 2 3 4 5 6 7
		Add 8 hours >		1 2 3 4 5 6 7
		Add 8 hours >		1 2 3 4 5 6 7
		Add 8 hours >		1 2 3 4 5 6 7

keto**CONTINUUM #6**

Date	TIME: First Bite or Sip (first calorie or sweeteners)		When you will stop all calories, chewing and sweeteners	How many days in a row did you make it?
		Add 8 hours >		1 2 3 4 5 6 7
		Add 8 hours >		1 2 3 4 5 6 7
		Add 8 hours >		1 2 3 4 5 6 7
		Add 8 hours >		1 2 3 4 5 6 7
		Add 8 hours >		1 2 3 4 5 6 7
		Add 8 hours >		1 2 3 4 5 6 7
		Add 8 hours >		1 2 3 4 5 6 7
		Add 8 hours >		1 2 3 4 5 6 7
		Add 8 hours >		1 2 3 4 5 6 7
		Add 8 hours >		1 2 3 4 5 6 7
		Add 8 hours >		1 2 3 4 5 6 7

4.5 KETOCONTINUUM #7

ketoCONTINUUM	GUIDELINES	NEXT STEPS
#7: 23:1 OMAD ALL in one hour	ALL calories and sweeteners in one hour. 23 hours = Only salt, water, tea or coffee.	Begin checking blood numbers right before you eat.

23 + 1 = 24 23:1
23:1 23 hours of fasting. 1 hour to eat.

OMAD: One Meal A Day
ACIOH: All calories in one hour

ketoCONTINUUM #7 provides the opportunity for psychological growth.
Mastering ketoCONTINUUM #6 best prepared you for the lessons you will learn at this stage. Once you have seven consecutive days limiting your calories to eight hours, use the charts in this section to track further progress on limiting your eating window. The far-right column offers 8 hours of eating. Shade in the number of hours from your first calorie to your last.

1		4		8

The goal is to limit it to one hour. Don't jump from eight hours of eating to one. This continuum takes time to master. Gradually limit your eating window. The shaded bars easily show your progress. The charts reveal patterns of your behavior. Be honest with your documentation. Then study your charts. This is critical to understanding yourself. I recommend sharing these charts with your accountability partner. Sometimes they see the patterns better.

When you find yourself at a number of hours that you can't seem to reduce further, stay there. Even though the goal is one hour, many people find enormous benefits in using a 4-hour eating window. That equation fits their current season of life better. As a result, they remain consistent and stay the course. That's a win!

	ketoCONTINUUM		WHO DOES THE WORK?	TEST
BEGINNER	#1:	I eat every 2–4 hours	CHEMISTRY CARRIES YOU	X
	#2:	LESS THAN 20 total carbs		Urine PeeTone Strips
	#3:	I "accidentally" missed a meal. [Keto-adapted]		
BASELINE METABOLISM	#4:	Eat 2 meals per day	YOU DO THE WORK. Discipline needed for each new step.	
	#5:	16:8		
	#6:	Advanced 16:8		
	#7:	23:1 OMAD ALL in one hour		
	#8:	Advanced 23:1/OMAD		Blood Ketone Strips
STRESSING METABOLISM	#9:	36-hour fast	PSYCHOLOGY. Use tribe for best results.	
	#10:	36-hour fast without a celebration meal		
	#11:	48-hour fast		
	#12:	72-hour fast		

	Wake Up Time	Morning STATS (Measure at routine times)			GOAL: Keep eating within the hours from 6 AM to 11 PM		GOAL: Reduce # of hours
		Glucose	Ketones	Dr. Boz Ratio	Eating Window Time Open	Eating Window Time Closed	# of Hours for Eating Window
WEEK ___							
SUN							1 4 8
MON							1 4 8
TUE							1 4 8
WED							1 4 8
THU							1 4 8
FRI							1 4 8
SAT							1 4 8
WEEK ___							
SUN							1 4 8
MON							1 4 8
TUE							1 4 8
WED							1 4 8
THU							1 4 8
FRI							1 4 8
SAT							1 4 8

KETOCONTINUUM #7

	Wake Up Time	Morning STATS (Measure at routine times)			GOAL: Keep eating within the hours from 6 AM to 11 PM		GOAL: Reduce # of hours
		Glucose	Ketones	Dr. Boz Ratio	Eating Window Time Open	Eating Window Time Closed	# of Hours for Eating Window
WEEK ___							
SUN							1 4 8
MON							1 4 8
TUE							1 4 8
WED							1 4 8
THU							1 4 8
FRI							1 4 8
SAT							1 4 8
WEEK ___							
SUN							1 4 8
MON							1 4 8
TUE							1 4 8
WED							1 4 8
THU							1 4 8
FRI							1 4 8
SAT							1 4 8

KETOCONTINUUM #7

| | Wake Up Time | Morning STATS (Measure at routine times) | | | GOAL: Keep eating within the hours from 6 AM to 11 PM | | GOAL: Reduce # of hours |
		Glucose	Ketones	Dr. Boz Ratio	Eating Window Time Open	Eating Window Time Closed	# of Hours for Eating Window
WEEK ___							
SUN							1 4 8
MON							1 4 8
TUE							1 4 8
WED							1 4 8
THU							1 4 8
FRI							1 4 8
SAT							1 4 8
WEEK ___							
SUN							1 4 8
MON							1 4 8
TUE							1 4 8
WED							1 4 8
THU							1 4 8
FRI							1 4 8
SAT							1 4 8

ketoCONTINUUM #7

	Wake Up Time	Morning STATS (Measure at routine times)			GOAL: Keep eating within the hours from 6 AM to 11 PM		GOAL: Reduce # of hours
	Wake Up Time	Glucose	Ketones	Dr. Boz Ratio	Eating Window Time Open	Eating Window Time Closed	# of Hours for Eating Window
WEEK ___							
SUN							1 4 8
MON							1 4 8
TUE							1 4 8
WED							1 4 8
THU							1 4 8
FRI							1 4 8
SAT							1 4 8
WEEK ___							
SUN							1 4 8
MON							1 4 8
TUE							1 4 8
WED							1 4 8
THU							1 4 8
FRI							1 4 8
SAT							1 4 8

KETOCONTINUUM #7

	Wake Up Time	Morning STATS (Measure at routine times)			GOAL: Keep eating within the hours from 6 AM to 11 PM		GOAL: Reduce # of hours
		Glucose	Ketones	Dr. Boz Ratio	Eating Window Time Open	Eating Window Time Closed	# of Hours for Eating Window
WEEK ___							
SUN							1 4 8
MON							1 4 8
TUE							1 4 8
WED							1 4 8
THU							1 4 8
FRI							1 4 8
SAT							1 4 8
WEEK ___							
SUN							1 4 8
MON							1 4 8
TUE							1 4 8
WED							1 4 8
THU							1 4 8
FRI							1 4 8
SAT							1 4 8

4.6 ketoCONTINUUM #8

ketoCONTINUUM	GUIDELINES	NEXT STEPS
#8: Advanced 23:1/OMAD	Move eating-hour within 11 hours following sunrise to match your circadian rhythm.	Record the Dr. Boz ratio first thing int he morning. Repeat before eating.

From this point forward, the charts span both the left and right pages of the workbook.

ketoCONTINUUM #8 reveals a great deal of information in the charts. Do not feel pressured to fill in every column every day. The chart provides space when you check metrics, but it's not expected that you measure all of these every day.

Use ketoCONTINUUM #8's chart to study the time you eating and sleep. Do your best to document your wake-up time and shade your hours of eating.

	Wake Up Time	Morning STATS (Measure at routine times)			Time you broke your fast	Hours Fasted	Break-Fast STATS (Measure right before eating/drinking your first calorie)		
		Glucose	Ketones	Dr. Boz Ratio			Break-Fast Glucose	Break-Fast Ketone	Break-Fast Dr Boz Ratio
WEEK ___									
SUN									
MON									
TUE									
WED									
THU									
FRI									
SAT									

The most valuable time to check your Dr. Boz Ratio is first thing in the morning. I suggest measuring it 3-5 times a week when you are trying to look for patterns of how your body is responding. Adding a measurement right before you break your fast has value, but not as much as your morning metrics.

I encourage students to work towards two goals in this section::

1) Keep your eating window the same number of hours as ketoCONTINUUM #7.
   If you found a 3-hour eating window optimal for this season of your life, stay there. Do your best not to lengthen the time from first bite to last bite.

2) Slide your hours of consumption towards sunrise. Your natural rise in cortisol surges at dawn and returns to baseline 4-6 hours later. This corresponds to a rise in blood sugar and therefore a rise in insulin. Eating also increases your insulin. Overlapping your morning rise in these hormones with your eating window offers a pattern that mimics fasting.
   Start by closing your eating window by 5 PM. Next, slide your hours of eating as close to sunrise as you can

GOAL: Keep eating window within the hours from 6 AM to 5 PM Shade the time your eating window opens to time it closes																GOAL: Keep # hours stable.
6 AM	7 AM	8 AM	9 AM	10 AM	11 AM	12 NOON	1 PM	2 PM	3 PM	4 PM	5 PM	6 PM	7 PM	8 PM	9 PM	# of Hours for Eating Window
																1 4 8
																1 4 8
																1 4 8
																1 4 8
																1 4 8
																1 4 8
																1 4 8

	Wake Up Time	Morning STATS (Measure at routine times)			Time you broke your fast	Hours Fasted	Break-Fast STATS (Measure right before eating/drinking your first calorie)		
		Glucose	Ketones	Dr. Boz Ratio			Break-Fast Glucose	Break-Fast Ketone	Break-Fast Dr Boz Ratio
WEEK ___									
SUN									
MON									
TUE									
WED									
THU									
FRI									
SAT									
WEEK ___									
SUN									
MON									
TUES									
WED									
THU									
FRI									
SAT									

ketoCONTINUUM Workbook

6 AM	7 AM	8 AM	9 AM	10 AM	11 AM	12 NOON	1 PM	2 PM	3 PM	4 PM	5 PM	# of Hours for Eating Window

GOAL: Keep eating window within the hours from 6 AM to 5 PM
Shade the time your eating window opens to time it closes

GOAL: Keep # hours stable.

1	4	8
1	4	8
1	4	8
1	4	8
1	4	8
1	4	8
1	4	8
1	4	8
1	4	8
1	4	8
1	4	8
1	4	8
1	4	8
1	4	8

	Wake Up Time	Morning STATS (Measure at routine times)			Time you broke your fast	Hours Fasted	Break-Fast STATS (Measure right before eating/drinking your first calorie)		
		Glucose	Ketones	Dr. Boz Ratio			Break-Fast Glucose	Break-Fast Ketone	Break-Fast Dr Boz Ratio
WEEK ___									
SUN									
MON									
TUE									
WED									
THU									
FRI									
SAT									
WEEK ___									
SUN									
MON									
TUES									
WED									
THU									
FRI									
SAT									

ketoCONTINUUM Workbook

GOAL: Keep eating window within the hours from 6 AM to 5 PM Shade the time your eating window opens to time it closes																GOAL: Keep # hours stable.
6 AM	7 AM	8 AM	9 AM	10 AM	11 AM	12 NOON	1 PM	2 PM	3 PM	4 PM	5 PM	6 PM	7 PM	8 PM	9 PM	# of Hours for Eating Window
																1 4 8
																1 4 8
																1 4 8
																1 4 8
																1 4 8
																1 4 8
																1 4 8
																1 4 8
																1 4 8
																1 4 8
																1 4 8
																1 4 8
																1 4 8
																1 4 8

	Wake Up Time	Morning STATS (Measure at routine times)			Time you broke your fast	Hours Fasted	Break-Fast STATS (Measure right before eating/drinking your first calorie)		
		Glucose	Ketones	Dr. Boz Ratio			Break-Fast Glucose	Break-Fast Ketone	Break-Fast Dr Boz Ratio
WEEK ___									
SUN									
MON									
TUE									
WED									
THU									
FRI									
SAT									
WEEK ___									
SUN									
MON									
TUES									
WED									
THU									
FRI									
SAT									

ketoCONTINUUM Workbook

																GOAL: Keep # hours stable.
GOAL: Keep eating window within the hours from 6 AM to 5 PM Shade the time your eating window opens to time it closes																
6 AM	7 AM	8 AM	9 AM	10 AM	11 AM	12 NOON	1 PM	2 PM	3 PM	4 PM	5 PM	6 PM	7 PM	8 PM	9 PM	# of Hours for Eating Window
																1 4 8
																1 4 8
																1 4 8
																1 4 8
																1 4 8
																1 4 8
																1 4 8
																1 4 8
																1 4 8
																1 4 8
																1 4 8
																1 4 8
																1 4 8
																1 4 8

SECTION

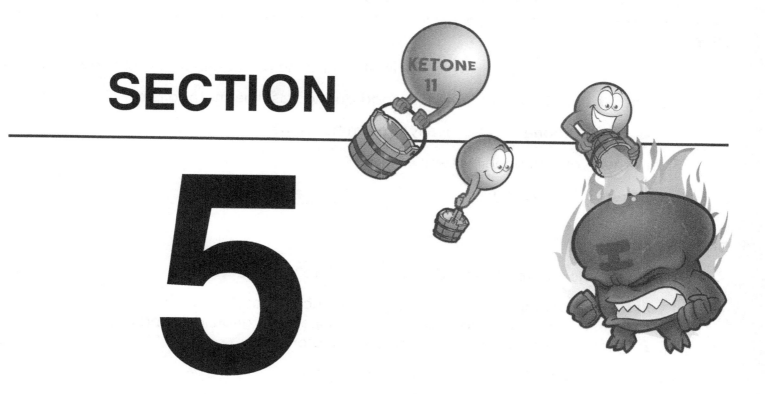

5

FASTING CYCLES

5.1   Overview of Fasting Cycles

5.2   ketoCONTINUUM #9 & #10

5.3   ketoCONTINUUM #11 & 12

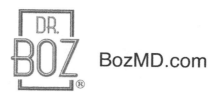

BozMD.com

5.1 OVERVIEW OF FASTING CYCLES

WHY?

- Advance your metabolism while living at a baseline metabolism that fits your life.

- Strengthen your ability to say no to food during baseline metabolisms.

- Pulse your hormones— specifically growth hormone.

- Strengthen your immune system.

- For advanced autophagy.

DO NOT FAST IF:

1. If you take blood pressure medication. Speak to your doctor first.

2. If you take medication to lower blood sugar such as insulin, sulfonylureas (glyburide, glimepiride, tolbutamide, chlorpropamide, glipizide), and many other diabetic medications. Speak to your doctor first.

3. If you take Coumadin, speak to your doctor first.

4. If you have not been at one of the baseline metabolisms for a minimum of two weeks, do not fast yet.

DRINKS DURING A FAST: GOOD, BETTER, BEST

GOOD:

Bone Broth: Be sure to add salt. The first dozen times I fasted, I drank bone broth whenever I craved something. Any whimsical thought of food led me to the trough for broth. A stingy amount of salt flavored every sip. Looking back, I struggled to let go of the comfort of food and I needed more salt. Each fast I "needed" less broth and I practiced new coping skills to comfort my stress. I also found solé water. Adding solé water sooner would have saved many of my struggles.

If you enjoy time in the kitchen, find my favorite bone broth recipe below. If you prefer to click and deliver, stick with Kettle & Fire. (Promo Code: DrBoz) on.bozmd.com/bonebroth

BETTER:

Ketones-in-a-Can: It only takes a pinch. During a fast, the slightest addition of ketones makes a dynamic difference. By this stage of the ketoCONTINUUM, your system knows how to use ketones. Fasting stresses your metabolism and demands more fuel. Increased ketones will flow from your liver's mitochondria in response to this mismatch between energy supply and demand. During the stress your fuel supply is low and you feel awful. Too much time spent in this mismatch can ruin a fast. Each fast your metabolism improves and the mismatch shortens. For the unseasoned faster, sipping on ketones can save the fast by bridging the gap. Sips of concentrated Ketones-in-a-Can boost circulating ketones in as little as 10 minutes.

If you feel yucky for longer than 40 minutes, break your fast. Forty minutes can feel like a lifetime during your first few fasts. Mix a tablespoon of powder in a small shot glass. Sip on it for 20 minutes. If nothing improves by 40 minutes, give up. Try again another day.

Black Coffee: This is my new favorite. During my formative fasts, I added heavy whipping cream to my coffee. I loved it. However, I failed to fast longer than 36 hours, and my Dr. Boz Ratio barely dropped. Removing the cream and adding solé water tipped me towards success. The perfect fast limits you to only water and salt. I have no interest in being perfect. Salty black coffee is good enough for me.

Tea: Tea offers another "better" choice while fasting. As I curb my coffee habit by substituting tea, my palate for tea is fragile. I don't like the taste of instant tea. Similarly, it only took one sip from molded tea leaves to ruin my budding attraction. Pique Tea restored my faith a bit. They freeze dry fresh tea leaves into crystals after making sure there are no extra chemicals in the plant's agriculture. It's the only way I drink tea now. on.bozmd.com/fast_with_tea

BEST:

Salt and water win the BEST title when fasting. This is also called a strict fast.

BONE BROTH THAT GELS EVERY SINGLE TIME

www.MeatButterEggs.com

PREP TIME: 5 MINS   **COOK TIME IN INSTANT POT:** 4 HOURS   **SERVINGS:** 8 CUPS

INGREDIENTS:

- 8 cups water: Measure the water. Do not fill your instant pot to the fill line. It's too much water.
- 2 whole chicken carcasses. Remove the meat and use the leftover bones. Your pot should be as full as you can get it.
- 1 package chicken feet (about 20 feet)
- 1 tsp salt

INSTRUCTIONS:

1. Throw bones, chicken feet, salt and water into your pot.
2. Using the soup function on your Instapot, set your time to 240 minutes. Make sure your valve is closed.
3. After 4 hours let the instant pot do a natural pressure release to avoid broth spraying all over your kitchen.
4. Strain through a cheesecloth into containers. Eat or let cool before chilling in the refrigerator overnight and then freezing what you won't use up that week.
5. Don't remove the fat off the top. It helps seal the broth and keeps it fresh.

INSTANT POT: This is a modern day pressure cooker. It is safer than the traditional pressure cookers and adds a variety of foods to the list.

BONES: Save the carcasses from rotisserie chicken in the freezer. When you have enough bones to fill your pot, make broth.

CHICKEN FEET: Don't leave out the feet. The collagen comes from the chicken feet. This makes your broth rich, flavorful and nutritionally dense. Using an instant pot, or a traditional pressure cooker, there is no need to blanch, skin or remove the nails. Just throw them all into the pot. There is no difference in taste or appearance.

*TIP: Save the carcasses of rotisserie chickens. Toss them in a plastic pail in the freezer until you accumulate three or four carcasses. This makes the best broth.

BREAKING A FAST: GOOD, BETTER, BEST

GOOD:

Simply eat a normal keto meal. WARNING: high amounts of carbs, high volume of food, or alcohol can cause quite the flush of diarrhea. A fast lasting longer than 48 hours turns off the secretion production that lubricates the lumen of your gut. Healthy mucus-producing cells store up their secretions normally expelled during fasting. Eating opens the flood gates to a wave of slimy lubrication for the gut. The end result: Diarrhea.

Keep it keto. Try not to overeat. Limit alcohol to one drink.

BETTER:

A better break-fast option is salty or fermented food thirty minutes before your meal. Kombucha (be sure the pH is less than 3.5) or salty bone broth works well. If I fast for 72 hours, I love a cold Pickle Juice Pop Cycle while I prepare the meal.

The salt or acidic substance releases some of the stored secretions from the mucus cells of the gut. After 30-60 minutes, feast on your favorite fatty meat before eating the other parts of the meal. Keep it as keto as you can. Avoid alcohol with this meal.

BEST:

Use the salty or fermented advice above. Give the gut a full hour before eating. BEST separates from better by way of the size of the meal. Eat a "normal" keto meal to break your fast. A celebration meal causes quite the dumping, even if led with salt or fermented food. Keep the size of the meal within reason for the best results.

ketoCONTINUUM #9: 36-HOUR-FAST

- Thirty-six hours is actually only one day. Yes. Not one and a half days— it's ONE DAY.

- Place the 36-hours without food over two nights of sleeping.

- Eight hours the first night plus eight hours the second night. Strategically place those 16 hours of fasting during sleep.

- That leaves only one day of fasting.

- Focus from one sunrise to sunset, that's all.

- Eat your evening meal as usual. Take note of the time of your final bite of food. That officially begins your fast. That evening plays out no differently than the past nights.

- Follow David's example from his first fast by tucking into bed as normal without sharing your fasting plan to anyone.

- "Head down. Mouth Shut." Vs. Share with a supportive Support Group. David approached his first fast in careful isolation. His household was nervous about him fasting. There was simply too much emotional baggage to carry if he shared his plans to fast. He succeeded by privately fasting the first few times. An alternate approach is to partner with supportive veteran fasters from your Keto Support Group. This is why a group exists — to support one another through times of struggle.

ketoCONTINUUM #10: 36-HOUR FAST WITHOUT CELEBRATION MEAL

After completing your first fast, the smell, taste, and joy of food feels delightful. Beware. Routine celebrations after a fast can blossom into an onerous pattern.

ketoCONTINUUM #11: 48-HOUR FAST

- Fits well into a schedule of OMAD. Even if your eating window is still 4 hours, I find this option easy to duplicate.

- Think of missing ONE MEAL. With strong keto adaption, this is not as awful as it sounds. One meal is missed.

- BEWARE: The first several times you do this, ketones soar on the second night. This makes it difficult to sleep. As your body practices this metabolic stress, your over-production of ketones fades.

ketoCONTINUUM #12: 72-HOUR FAST

One 72-hour fast every week for eight consecutive weeks marks an excellent badge of pride and accomplishment. The remaining four days of the week, return to your preferred baseline metabolism. This stressor delivers on these promises:

- Empties glycogen

- Spikes growth hormone

- Ramps up norepinephrine

- Triggers autophagy

- Unlocks the gift of fasting for a lifetime

	# Hours Fasting	Difficulty Level 1-5	Metabolic Stress Level 1-5	Advantages	Challenges
36 Hours	36	1	2	Significant metabolic improvement with 1 day & 2 nights.	The first one is the hardest. Once you break through the mental barrier, this gets easier.
36 Hours Without Celebration Meal	36	2	2	The metabolic stress is the same as the 36-hour fast. The NO CELEBRATION skill is critical for advanced ketosis.	Celebration meals are closely linked to struggles with food addiction.
48 Hours	48	2	3	Works well for those who eat primary meals with other non-fasters. The mealtime schedule stays the same. You miss only one shared meal.	The first one is the hardest.
1:47 OMEOD	47	3	4	Eight weeks of this pattern reverses many chronic issues. The natural rise in ketones is beautifully demonstrated with this option.	The difficulty of 1:47 OMEOD grows with time. Social isolation becomes a major obstacle. For best results, find a partner. RECOMMENDATIONS: check-ins with accountability partner & substitute non-eating activity during mealtime.
Calorie Restricted OMAD 23:1	23	5	5	This fasting protocol is added to oncology regimes for some of the deadliest cancers. Caloric restriction of 500 calories creates a powerful shift in energy resources.	Do not be deceived by the short fasting time. Limiting intake to 500 calories proves extremely challenging. Do not do this without supervision. Must use Cronometer App! Essential nutrients must be monitored.
Two Months of Weekly 72 Hour Fasts	72	4	4	Growth hormone soars when fasting 72-hours in addition to ketoCONTINUUM #6-#8. Eight consecutive weeks reverses setbacks, eliminates weight loss stalls, erases a majority of chronic inflammation, and unlocks the ultimate fasting tool for a lifetime	The first one is the hardest. Do not attempt until you've lived at baseline metabolism for at least 2 weeks. If you have been fasting in secret, 72-hours is not "hide able."

I have listed three patterns of eating that significantly advance metabolisms. In my clinical practice, our team works very closely with keto-adapted patients who use these. We do not advance to these options until patients have mastered the ability to remove all calories from 20 hours of their day. The absence of intake for most of the hours of the day must be routine before advancing to these metabolic stressors.

1. **1:47 OMEOD: One Meal Every Other Day.** To clarify, that's one satiating meal followed by 47 hours of fasting for two months.

OMEOD offers a pattern of eating with one meal every other day. Like ketoCONTINUUM #8 [Advanced 23:1], the benefit of a predictable schedule teases many to try this. Indeed, this stress rapidly improves metabolism. Eating one satiating meal every Monday, Wednesday, Friday, and Saturday provides a pattern where some people flourish. However, the drawbacks show up in the weeks that follow. This schedule wears on people. They find themselves isolated from loved ones who can't follow such a strict regime. The isolation away from the social part of eating seems tolerable at first. Ironically, it is often the hunger for the relationships that cracks their persistence as opposed to hunger for food. Social isolation breaks them down. OMEAD improves metabolism without fail. Beware of the consequences to your relationships.

2. **CALORIE RESTRICTED OMAD 23:1.** For 2 months limit consumption to less than 900 kcal (in some cases 500 kcal) in your solitary daily ketogenic meal.

Decreasing caloric intake while using ketoCONTINUUM #8 intensely stresses metabolism. With fat-based hormones in full supply, autophagy sweeps through your cellular health. The protocol added to deadly cancer regimes further limits calories from 900 kcal to 500 kcal per day. These teams carefully supervise their patients' progress as they race against time. This protocol is intense and requires careful medical supervision with the sickest audience of patients. Outside of this crisis, consider the 900 kcal limit for a goal of two months. This extremely lofty goal provides a very intense workout for your metabolism.

3. Eight consecutive weeks of ketoCONTINUUM #12: 72-hour fast

"Doc, how long does it take to empty the glycogen bubbles from my liver?"
Answer: "It depends upon the size of your liver and the state of your chemistry."

I encourage students to use this third metabolic stressor to break through a plateau in their progress. This metabolic stressor easily fits into many people's lives without the dangerous risks listed above. By the end of the eight consecutive weeks, many have resumed their desired weight loss, decreased their pain, or lowered their medication for chronic disease. At the end of eight weeks, students universally appreciate how much easier it is to say, "No thank you" to food. This gift lasts a lifetime.

5.2 KETOCONTINUUM #9 & #10

ketoCONTINUUM	GUIDELINES	NEXT STEPS
#9: 36-hour fast	Fast for 36 hours. No calories. No sweeteners. Start in evening as to use 2 cycles of sleep during the 36 hours.	Begin fast after evening meal. DANGER: If on blood pressure meds or blood sugar lowing meds. ASK YOUR DOCTOR.
#10: 36-hour fast without a celebration meal	After 36-hour fast, return to your normal pattern of eating without a splurge meal.	Offer a group fasting routine to others in your tribe. Fast together.

Welcome to fasting.

I recommend adding a fast to any of the baseline metabolisms. Consider ketoCONTINUUMs #5-#8 your cardio-workouts for your mitochondria and fasting as your strength-training.

Like the previous section, the chart on the left page tracks your DBR first thing in the morning and offers a measurement prior to breaking your fast.

Reminder: the morning metrics best reflect your body's health. If you're only going to check one set of numbers, choose that one.

Use the chart on the following page to track your first dozen fasts. Paying attention to the items in this chart will help you succeed at fasting. Before each fast, set a goal. Document the number of hours you want to fast and the options you plan to use if you need a crutch.

Personally, I also write down what I will pray for during times of struggle. Fasting and prayer enhance each other. When I have properly prepared for a fast, I succeed. When I don't have my goal in mind, don't have a backup plan during a difficult transition, or don't have a specific prayer in mind, I fail. Similarly, if I plan my break-fasting meal during my hours of fasting, it's often a gluttonous meal. Prevent that overindulgence by planning how you will break your fast before you start.

The charts on the following pages are designed to use on fasting and non-fasting days. Notice the hours on the right page span the full day. Track the hours of fasting overnight and into the following day. Document the foods you eat over the time you eat.

Work to keep your eating window as narrow as possible. Notice the patterns that happen after a fast. What were your numbers the day following a fast? How much worse were they if you binged or celebrated after your fast?

	ketoCONTINUUM	WHO DOES THE WORK?	TEST
BEGINNER	**#1:** I eat every 2–4 hours	CHEMISTRY CARRIES YOU	X
	#2: LESS THAN 20 total carbs		Urine PeeTone Strips
	#3: I "accidentally" missed a meal. [Keto-adapted]		
BASELINE METABOLISM	**#4:** Eat 2 meals per day	YOU DO THE WORK. Discipline needed for each new step.	
	#5: 16:8		
	#6: Advanced 16:8		
	#7: 23:1 OMAD ALL in one hour		
	#8: Advanced 23:1/OMAD		
STRESSING METABOLISM	**#9:** 36-hour fast	PSYCHOLOGY. Use tribe for best results.	Blood Ketone Strips
	#10: 36-hour fast without a celebration meal		
	#11: 48-hour fast		
	#12: 72-hour fast		

Date	Goal For Fast	Hours Fasted	Did you use a crutch?	What did you consume during your fast? (Water, bone broth, BHB, coffee, keto-coffee, solé water)	How did you break your fast?
			Yes No		
			Yes No		
			Yes No		
			Yes No		
			Yes No		
			Yes No		
			Yes No		
			Yes No		
			Yes No		
			Yes No		
			Yes No		
			Yes No		

	Morning STATS (Measure at routine time)			Break-Fast STATS (Measure right before eating/ drinking your first calorie)			TIME: Last Bite / Calorie	TIME: First Bite/ Calorie that Broke the Fast	Total Hours Fasted
	Glucose	Ketones	Dr. Boz Ratio	Break-Fast Glucose	Break-Fast Ketones	Break-Fast Dr Boz Ratio			
WEEK ____									
SUN									
MON									
TUE									
WED									
THU									
FRI									
SAT									
WEEK ____									
SUN									
MON									
TUES									
WED									
THU									
FRI									
SAT									

ketoCONTINUUM Workbook

															GOAL: Resume Your Standard Window
GOAL: Find a rhythm for fasting. Track your numbers. Watch for patterns that lead to success and those that predict a stumble.															
6-7 AM	8 AM	9 AM	10-11 AM	12 Noon	1-2 PM	3-4 PM	5 PM	6 PM	7 PM	8 PM	9 PM	10 PM	11-12 Mid night	1-5 AM	# of Hours for Eating Window
															1 4 8
															1 4 8
															1 4 8
															1 4 8
															1 4 8
															1 4 8
															1 4 8
															1 4 8
															1 4 8
															1 4 8
															1 4 8
															1 4 8
															1 4 8
															1 4 8

	Morning STATS (Measure at routine time)			Break-Fast STATS (Measure right before eating/ drinking your first calorie)			TIME: Last Bite / Calorie	TIME: First Bite/ Calorie that Broke the Fast	Total Hours Fasted
	Glucose	Ketones	Dr. Boz Ratio	Break-Fast Glucose	Break-Fast Ketones	Break-Fast Dr Boz Ratio			
WEEK ____									
SUN									
MON									
TUE									
WED									
THU									
FRI									
SAT									
WEEK ____									
SUN									
MON									
TUES									
WED									
THU									
FRI									
SAT									

ketoCONTINUUM Workbook

															GOAL: Resume Your Standard Window
\multicolumn{16}{c}{GOAL: Find a rhythm for fasting. Track your numbers. Watch for patterns that lead to success and those that predict a stumble.}

6-7 AM	8 AM	9 AM	10-11 AM	12 Noon	1-2 PM	3-4 PM	5 PM	6 PM	7 PM	8 PM	9 PM	10 PM	11-12 Mid night	1-5 AM	# of Hours for Eating Window
															1 4 8
															1 4 8
															1 4 8
															1 4 8
															1 4 8
															1 4 8
															1 4 8
															1 4 8
															1 4 8
															1 4 8
															1 4 8
															1 4 8
															1 4 8
															1 4 8

	Morning STATS (Measure at routine time)			Break-Fast STATS (Measure right before eating/ drinking your first calorie)			TIME: Last Bite / Calorie	TIME: First Bite/ Calorie that Broke the Fast	Total Hours Fasted
	Glucose	Ketones	Dr. Boz Ratio	Break-Fast Glucose	Break-Fast Ketones	Break-Fast Dr Boz Ratio			
WEEK ____									
SUN									
MON									
TUE									
WED									
THU									
FRI									
SAT									
WEEK ____									
SUN									
MON									
TUES									
WED									
THU									
FRI									
SAT									

ketoCONTINUUM Workbook

															GOAL: Resume Your Standard Window

GOAL: Find a rhythm for fasting.
Track your numbers. Watch for patterns that lead to success and those that predict a stumble.

6-7 AM	8 AM	9 AM	10-11 AM	12 Noon	1-2 PM	3-4 PM	5 PM	6 PM	7 PM	8 PM	9 PM	10 PM	11-12 Mid night	1-5 AM	# of Hours for Eating Window
															1 4 8
															1 4 8
															1 4 8
															1 4 8
															1 4 8
															1 4 8
															1 4 8
															1 4 8
															1 4 8
															1 4 8
															1 4 8
															1 4 8
															1 4 8
															1 4 8

	Morning STATS (Measure at routine time)			Break-Fast STATS (Measure right before eating/ drinking your first calorie)			TIME: Last Bite / Calorie	TIME: First Bite/ Calorie that Broke the Fast	Total Hours Fasted
	Glucose	Ketones	Dr. Boz Ratio	Break-Fast Glucose	Break-Fast Ketones	Break-Fast Dr Boz Ratio			
WEEK ____									
SUN									
MON									
TUE									
WED									
THU									
FRI									
SAT									
WEEK ____									
SUN									
MON									
TUES									
WED									
THU									
FRI									
SAT									

ketoCONTINUUM Workbook

GOAL: Find a rhythm for fasting. Track your numbers. Watch for patterns that lead to success and those that predict a stumble.															GOAL: Resume Your Standard Window
6-7 AM	8 AM	9 AM	10-11 AM	12 Noon	1-2 PM	3-4 PM	5 PM	6 PM	7 PM	8 PM	9 PM	10 PM	11-12 Mid night	1-5 AM	# of Hours for Eating Window
															1 4 8
															1 4 8
															1 4 8
															1 4 8
															1 4 8
															1 4 8
															1 4 8
															1 4 8
															1 4 8
															1 4 8
															1 4 8
															1 4 8
															1 4 8
															1 4 8

5.3 KETOCONTINUUM #11 & 12

ketoCONTINUUM	GUIDELINES	NEXT STEPS
#11: 48-hour fast	Fast for 48 hours. No calories. No sweeteners.	Safe to try twice a week. Unlike the 36-hour fast, this option keeps meals at the same time each day.
#12: 72-hour fast	Fast for 72 hours. No calories. No Sweeteners.	When the timing is right, stress your metabolism with 8 weeks of a 72-hour fast. The rest of the week, return to your BASELINE METABOLISM. The best transitions happen through this challenge.

This section's chart matches Section 5.2. Lengthening your fast beyond 36 hours often happens naturally by the third or fourth fast.

Continue to add your consumed foods to the right page while documenting your blood biomarkers on the left.

Use the chart on the next page to summarize your first dozen longer fasts. Fill out this chart as you go. This documentation will reveal how to avoid repeat misstepped.

Prioritize checking your Dr. Boz Ratio twice on the final day of your fast. On that final day of your fast, the morning DBR is the most important measurement. The morning DBR reflects the rate of improvement against insulin resistance. Each fast allows a peek inside your mitochondria's health by measuring the morning DBR on the final day of the fast. Don't skip that measurement. When studying the health of patients, I follow this specific DBR to predict the rate of healing deep within their cells. Measure your fasting success by the improvements seen in this specific metric.

Approach the longer fasts with a specific prayer or mindfulness during the difficult minutes. Waiting for the emotional storm before you try to focus your thoughts invites failure. Write down where you will focus your thoughts BEFORE the fast begins.

After 48 or 72 hours of fasting, the way you break your fast becomes important. Diarrhea can be troublesome the first few times. Review the suggestions in Section 5.1 and document the complications such as cramping or diarrhea after eating.

	ketoCONTINUUM	WHO DOES THE WORK?	TEST
BEGINNER	**#1:** I eat every 2–4 hours	CHEMISTRY CARRIES YOU	X
	#2: LESS THAN 20 total carbs		Urine PeeTone Strips
	#3: I "accidentally" missed a meal. [Keto-adapted]		
BASELINE METABOLISM	**#4:** Eat 2 meals per day	YOU DO THE WORK. Discipline needed for each new step.	
	#5: 16:8		
	#6: Advanced 16:8		
	#7: 23:1 OMAD ALL in one hour		
	#8: Advanced 23:1/OMAD		Blood Ketone Strips
STRESSING METABOLISM	**#9:** 36-hour fast	PSYCHOLOGY. Use tribe for best results.	
	#10: 36-hour fast without a celebration meal		
	#11: 48-hour fast		
	#12: 72-hour fast		

Date	Goal For Fast (Hours + Mindfulness /Prayer Focus)	Hours Fasted	Did you use a crutch (Bone broth, BHB, Keto-coffee)		AM Dr. Boz Ratio the final day of fast	Break-Fast Dr Boz Ratio	How did you break your fast?	Complications after breaking fast
			Yes	No				
			Yes	No				
			Yes	No				
			Yes	No				
			Yes	No				
			Yes	No				
			Yes	No				
			Yes	No				
			Yes	No				
			Yes	No				
			Yes	No				
			Yes	No				

	Morning STATS (Measure at routine time)			Break-Fast STATS (Measure right before eating/ drinking your first calorie)			TIME: Last Bite / Calorie	TIME: First Bite/ Calorie that Broke the Fast	Total Hours Fasted
	Glucose	Ketones	Dr. Boz Ratio	Break-Fast Glucose	Break-Fast Ketones	Break-Fast Dr Boz Ratio			
WEEK ____									
SUN									
MON									
TUE									
WED									
THU									
FRI									
SAT									
WEEK ____									
SUN									
MON									
TUES									
WED									
THU									
FRI									
SAT									

ketoCONTINUUM Workbook

															GOAL: Resume Your Standard Window
GOAL: Find a rhythm for fasting. Track your numbers. Watch for patterns that lead to success and those that predict a stumble.															
6-7 AM	8 AM	9 AM	10-11 AM	12 Noon	1-2 PM	3-4 PM	5 PM	6 PM	7 PM	8 PM	9 PM	10 PM	11-12 Mid night	1-5 AM	# of Hours for Eating Window
															1 4 8
															1 4 8
															1 4 8
															1 4 8
															1 4 8
															1 4 8
															1 4 8
															1 4 8
															1 4 8
															1 4 8
															1 4 8
															1 4 8
															1 4 8
															1 4 8

	Morning STATS (Measure at routine time)			Break-Fast STATS (Measure right before eating/ drinking your first calorie)			TIME: Last Bite / Calorie	TIME: First Bite/ Calorie that Broke the Fast	Total Hours Fasted
	Glucose	Ketones	Dr. Boz Ratio	Break-Fast Glucose	Break-Fast Ketones	Break-Fast Dr Boz Ratio			
WEEK ___									
SUN									
MON									
TUE									
WED									
THU									
FRI									
SAT									
WEEK ___									
SUN									
MON									
TUES									
WED									
THU									
FRI									
SAT									

ketoCONTINUUM Workbook

															GOAL: Resume Your Standard Window
GOAL: Find a rhythm for fasting. Track your numbers. Watch for patterns that lead to success and those that predict a stumble.															
6-7 AM	8 AM	9 AM	10-11 AM	12 Noon	1-2 PM	3-4 PM	5 PM	6 PM	7 PM	8 PM	9 PM	10 PM	11-12 Mid night	1-5 AM	# of Hours for Eating Window
															1 4 8
															1 4 8
															1 4 8
															1 4 8
															1 4 8
															1 4 8
															1 4 8
															1 4 8
															1 4 8
															1 4 8
															1 4 8
															1 4 8
															1 4 8
															1 4 8

	Morning STATS (Measure at routine time)			Break-Fast STATS (Measure right before eating/ drinking your first calorie)			TIME: Last Bite / Calorie	TIME: First Bite/ Calorie that Broke the Fast	Total Hours Fasted
	Glucose	Ketones	Dr. Boz Ratio	Break-Fast Glucose	Break-Fast Ketones	Break-Fast Dr Boz Ratio			
WEEK ___									
SUN									
MON									
TUE									
WED									
THU									
FRI									
SAT									
WEEK ___									
SUN									
MON									
TUES									
WED									
THU									
FRI									
SAT									

ketoCONTINUUM Workbook

GOAL: Find a rhythm for fasting. Track your numbers. Watch for patterns that lead to success and those that predict a stumble.															GOAL: Resume Your Standard Window
6-7 AM	8 AM	9 AM	10-11 AM	12 Noon	1-2 PM	3-4 PM	5 PM	6 PM	7 PM	8 PM	9 PM	10 PM	11-12 Mid night	1-5 AM	# of Hours for Eating Window
															1 4 8
															1 4 8
															1 4 8
															1 4 8
															1 4 8
															1 4 8
															1 4 8
															1 4 8
															1 4 8
															1 4 8
															1 4 8
															1 4 8
															1 4 8
															1 4 8

	Morning STATS (Measure at routine time)			Break-Fast STATS (Measure right before eating/ drinking your first calorie)			TIME: Last Bite / Calorie	TIME: First Bite/ Calorie that Broke the Fast	Total Hours Fasted
	Glucose	Ketones	Dr. Boz Ratio	Break-Fast Glucose	Break-Fast Ketones	Break-Fast Dr Boz Ratio			
WEEK ___									
SUN									
MON									
TUE									
WED									
THU									
FRI									
SAT									
WEEK ___									
SUN									
MON									
TUES									
WED									
THU									
FRI									
SAT									

ketoCONTINUUM Workbook

															GOAL: Resume Your Standard Window

GOAL: Find a rhythm for fasting.
Track your numbers. Watch for patterns that lead to success
and those that predict a stumble.

6-7 AM	8 AM	9 AM	10-11 AM	12 Noon	1-2 PM	3-4 PM	5 PM	6 PM	7 PM	8 PM	9 PM	10 PM	11-12 Mid night	1-5 AM	# of Hours for Eating Window
															1 4 8
															1 4 8
															1 4 8
															1 4 8
															1 4 8
															1 4 8
															1 4 8
															1 4 8
															1 4 8
															1 4 8
															1 4 8
															1 4 8
															1 4 8
															1 4 8

	Morning STATS (Measure at routine time)			Break-Fast STATS (Measure right before eating/ drinking your first calorie)			TIME: Last Bite / Calorie	TIME: First Bite/ Calorie that Broke the Fast	Total Hours Fasted
	Glucose	Ketones	Dr. Boz Ratio	Break-Fast Glucose	Break-Fast Ketones	Break-Fast Dr Boz Ratio			
WEEK ____									
SUN									
MON									
TUE									
WED									
THU									
FRI									
SAT									
WEEK ____									
SUN									
MON									
TUES									
WED									
THU									
FRI									
SAT									

ketoCONTINUUM Workbook

GOAL: Find a rhythm for fasting. Track your numbers. Watch for patterns that lead to success and those that predict a stumble.															GOAL: Resume Your Standard Window
6-7 AM	8 AM	9 AM	10-11 AM	12 Noon	1-2 PM	3-4 PM	5 PM	6 PM	7 PM	8 PM	9 PM	10 PM	11-12 Mid night	1-5 AM	# of Hours for Eating Window
															1 4 8
															1 4 8
															1 4 8
															1 4 8
															1 4 8
															1 4 8
															1 4 8
															1 4 8
															1 4 8
															1 4 8
															1 4 8
															1 4 8
															1 4 8
															1 4 8

	Morning STATS (Measure at routine time)			Break-Fast STATS (Measure right before eating/ drinking your first calorie)			TIME: Last Bite / Calorie	TIME: First Bite/ Calorie that Broke the Fast	Total Hours Fasted
	Glucose	Ketones	Dr. Boz Ratio	Break-Fast Glucose	Break-Fast Ketones	Break-Fast Dr Boz Ratio			
WEEK ____									
SUN									
MON									
TUE									
WED									
THU									
FRI									
SAT									
WEEK ____									
SUN									
MON									
TUES									
WED									
THU									
FRI									
SAT									

ketoCONTINUUM Workbook

															GOAL: Resume Your Standard Window
GOAL: Find a rhythm for fasting. Track your numbers. Watch for patterns that lead to success and those that predict a stumble.															
6-7 AM	8 AM	9 AM	10-11 AM	12 Noon	1-2 PM	3-4 PM	5 PM	6 PM	7 PM	8 PM	9 PM	10 PM	11-12 Mid night	1-5 AM	# of Hours for Eating Window
															1 4 8
															1 4 8
															1 4 8
															1 4 8
															1 4 8
															1 4 8
															1 4 8
															1 4 8
															1 4 8
															1 4 8
															1 4 8
															1 4 8
															1 4 8
															1 4 8

	Morning STATS (Measure at routine time)			Break-Fast STATS (Measure right before eating/ drinking your first calorie)			TIME: Last Bite / Calorie	TIME: First Bite/ Calorie that Broke the Fast	Total Hours Fasted
	Glucose	Ketones	Dr. Boz Ratio	Break-Fast Glucose	Break-Fast Ketones	Break-Fast Dr Boz Ratio			
WEEK ____									
SUN									
MON									
TUE									
WED									
THU									
FRI									
SAT									
WEEK ____									
SUN									
MON									
TUES									
WED									
THU									
FRI									
SAT									

GOAL: Find a rhythm for fasting. Track your numbers. Watch for patterns that lead to success and those that predict a stumble.															GOAL: Resume Your Standard Window
6-7 AM	8 AM	9 AM	10-11 AM	12 Noon	1-2 PM	3-4 PM	5 PM	6 PM	7 PM	8 PM	9 PM	10 PM	11-12 Mid night	1-5 AM	# of Hours for Eating Window
															1　　4　　8
															1　　4　　8
															1　　4　　8
															1　　4　　8
															1　　4　　8
															1　　4　　8
															1　　4　　8
															1　　4　　8
															1　　4　　8
															1　　4　　8
															1　　4　　8
															1　　4　　8
															1　　4　　8
															1　　4　　8

	Morning STATS (Measure at routine time)			Break-Fast STATS (Measure right before eating/ drinking your first calorie)			TIME: Last Bite / Calorie	TIME: First Bite/ Calorie that Broke the Fast	Total Hours Fasted
	Glucose	Ketones	Dr. Boz Ratio	Break-Fast Glucose	Break-Fast Ketones	Break-Fast Dr Boz Ratio			
WEEK ____									
SUN									
MON									
TUE									
WED									
THU									
FRI									
SAT									
WEEK ____									
SUN									
MON									
TUES									
WED									
THU									
FRI									
SAT									

ketoCONTINUUM Workbook

															GOAL: Resume Your Standard Window
6-7 AM	8 AM	9 AM	10-11 AM	12 Noon	1-2 PM	3-4 PM	5 PM	6 PM	7 PM	8 PM	9 PM	10 PM	11-12 Mid night	1-5 AM	# of Hours for Eating Window
															1 4 8
															1 4 8
															1 4 8
															1 4 8
															1 4 8
															1 4 8
															1 4 8
															1 4 8
															1 4 8
															1 4 8
															1 4 8
															1 4 8
															1 4 8
															1 4 8

GOAL: Find a rhythm for fasting.
Track your numbers. Watch for patterns that lead to success
and those that predict a stumble.

	Morning STATS (Measure at routine time)			Break-Fast STATS (Measure right before eating/ drinking your first calorie)			TIME: Last Bite / Calorie	TIME: First Bite/ Calorie that Broke the Fast	Total Hours Fasted
	Glucose	Ketones	Dr. Boz Ratio	Break-Fast Glucose	Break-Fast Ketones	Break-Fast Dr Boz Ratio			
WEEK ____									
SUN									
MON									
TUE									
WED									
THU									
FRI									
SAT									
WEEK ____									
SUN									
MON									
TUES									
WED									
THU									
FRI									
SAT									

ketoCONTINUUM Workbook

GOAL: Find a rhythm for fasting. Track your numbers. Watch for patterns that lead to success and those that predict a stumble.															GOAL: Resume Your Standard Window
6-7 AM	8 AM	9 AM	10-11 AM	12 Noon	1-2 PM	3-4 PM	5 PM	6 PM	7 PM	8 PM	9 PM	10 PM	11-12 Mid night	1-5 AM	# of Hours for Eating Window
															1 4 8
															1 4 8
															1 4 8
															1 4 8
															1 4 8
															1 4 8
															1 4 8
															1 4 8
															1 4 8
															1 4 8
															1 4 8
															1 4 8
															1 4 8
															1 4 8

	Morning STATS (Measure at routine time)			Break-Fast STATS (Measure right before eating/ drinking your first calorie)			TIME: Last Bite / Calorie	TIME: First Bite/ Calorie that Broke the Fast	Total Hours Fasted
	Glucose	Ketones	Dr. Boz Ratio	Break-Fast Glucose	Break-Fast Ketones	Break-Fast Dr Boz Ratio			
WEEK ____									
SUN									
MON									
TUE									
WED									
THU									
FRI									
SAT									
WEEK ____									
SUN									
MON									
TUES									
WED									
THU									
FRI									
SAT									

ketoCONTINUUM Workbook

															GOAL: Resume Your Standard Window
6-7 AM	8 AM	9 AM	10-11 AM	12 Noon	1-2 PM	3-4 PM	5 PM	6 PM	7 PM	8 PM	9 PM	10 PM	11-12 Mid night	1-5 AM	# of Hours for Eating Window
															1 4 8
															1 4 8
															1 4 8
															1 4 8
															1 4 8
															1 4 8
															1 4 8
															1 4 8
															1 4 8
															1 4 8
															1 4 8
															1 4 8
															1 4 8
															1 4 8

GOAL: Find a rhythm for fasting. Track your numbers. Watch for patterns that lead to success and those that predict a stumble.

															GOAL: Resume Your Standard Window
6-7 AM	8 AM	9 AM	10-11 AM	12 Noon	1-2 PM	3-4 PM	5 PM	6 PM	7 PM	8 PM	9 PM	10 PM	11-12 Mid night	1-5 AM	# of Hours for Eating Window

GOAL: Find a rhythm for fasting.
Track your numbers. Watch for patterns that lead to success and those that predict a stumble.

1 4 8

1 4 8

1 4 8

1 4 8

1 4 8

1 4 8

1 4 8

1 4 8

1 4 8

1 4 8

1 4 8

1 4 8

1 4 8

1 4 8

ketoCONTINUUM

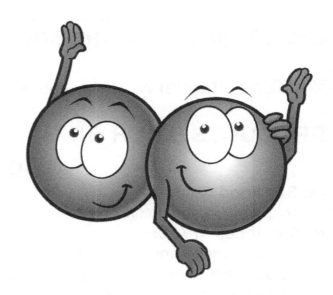

COMPILED RESOURCES

Links Throughout the Book

Charts

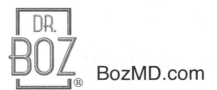

BozMD.com

LINKS THROUGHOUT THE BOOK

YouTube Playlist All Things Keto bit.ly/2yE1Caw

PRODUCTS BY DR BOZ-
<u>BozMD.com</u>

Dr. Boz Food Guide-
>   http://on.bozmd.com/FoodGuide

BHB Ketones-In-A-Can
- Raspberry Lemonade: http://on.bozmd.com/BHB1
- Cucumber Lemon: http://on.bozmd.com/BHB2
- Mexican Chocolate Spice: http://on.bozmd.com/BHB3
- Dutch Chocolate: http://on.bozmd.com/BHB4

Ketones-In-A-Capsule:
>   on.bozmd.com/BHBpill

Medium Chain Triglycerides C8:C10 Oil:
>   http://on.bozmd.com/c8c10

Dr. Boz Keto Combo
>   https://amzn.to/30jeL8w

Sleep Lecture by Dr. Boz
>   http://on.bozmd.com/sleep

Sleep Handout
>   http://on.bozmd.com/sleepHO

Cronometer: http://shrsl.com/24ok8

FORACARE - promo code: DrBoz

Meter FORACARE: http://on.bozmd.com/fora6
Thermometer: https://bit.ly/3beeaa7
Pulse Ox: http://on.bozmd.com/pulseox

PIQUE TEAS promo code DrBoz

Fermented Tea: http://on.bozmd.com/teas
Bergamot Fasting Tea: http://on.bozmd.com/BlackTea
Fast With Tea: http://on.bozmd.com/fast_with_tea

KETTLE & FIRE   promo code DrBoz

Beef & Chicken Bundle: http://on.bozmd.com/bonebroth
Chicken Broth: http://on.bozmd.com/chickenbroth
Beef Broth: http://on.bozmd.com/beefbroth
Keto Soup: http://on.bozmd.com/ketosoup

REDMONDS SALT- promo code Dr.Boz

Sucking Salt Rocks: http://bit.ly/3bkpZMl
Salt Refill: https://bit.ly/3dOdJFs
6-Pack Pocket Salt: http://bit.ly/31ypeen
Unflavored ReLytes: https://bit.ly/3evrhFe
Lemon ReLyte: https://bit.ly/3euE8aE
Licorice EarthPowder: https://bit.ly/3gmzD3r
BUCKET O' BENTONITE CLAY: https://bit.ly/2WCELbD
Jar of Bentonite Clay: https://bit.ly/32BkMOq

HOME A1C TESTING: https://amzn.to/37eg0b5

KETO PERFECT:

PERFECT KETO: http://bit.ly/2Q7BRtx
Choc Collagen: http://bit.ly/2EjnKfg
KETO COFFEE INSTANT: http://bit.ly/2RdLg3g
MCT Oil http://bit.ly/2Qzvvn5
Nut Butter: https://bit.ly/33kNHGM

OMEGA QUANT

Omega 3 Index http://on.bozmd.com/Omega3
Vitamin D Test: http://on.bozmd.com/vitD

MUSE HEADBAND:

MUSE: https://mbsy.co/muse/DrBoz

CHARTS

ketoCONTINUUM	Date									
1. I eat every 2–4 hours										
2. LESS THAN 20 total carbs										
3. I "accidentally" missed a meal. [Keto-adapted]										
4. Eat 2 meals per day										
5. 16:8										
6. Advanced 16:8										
7. 23:1 OMAD ALL in one hour										
8. Advanced 23:1/OMAD										
9. 36-hour fast										
10. 36-hour fast without a celebration meal										
11. 48-hour fast										
12. 72-hour fast										

THREE DAY CARB COUNT BEFORE YOU START CHART

Date	Food Diary before you change anything	Total Carbs
	Day 1	
	Day2	
	Day 3	

MEASUREMENT CHART

Date	Blood Pressure	BMI	Morning Fasting Glucose	Waistline	Neck Circumference	Thumb Shin-Print		Skin Tags
	<130/85	<25	<100	<40 in <35 in	<17 in	None		0

ketoCONTINUUM Workbook

LABORATORY CHART

Date	HgA1c	Omega 3 Index	Trans Fat Index	Vit D-25 Hydroxy	ALT	hsCRP	Uric Acid	CAC	Ferritin	TG/HDL mg/dl (mmol/L)
	<5.0 %	>8%	<1%	>50 ng/mL	<40u/L	<1.0 mg/L	<5.0 mg/ dL	<100	>50 ng/mL	<1.5 (<0.65)

ketoCONTINUUM ROADMAP

	ketoCONTINUUM	WHO DOES THE WORK?	TEST	GUIDELINES	NEXT STEPS	
BEGINNER	**#1:** I eat every 2–4 hours	CHEMISTRY CARRIES YOU	X	Fueled on glucose. Must refuel often. Never fueled by ketones.		4–6 WEEKS
	#2: I eat every 6–8 hours LESS THAN 20 total carbs		Urine PeeTone Strips	Eat <20 total carbs per day. Ketosis begins. Fat-based hormones rise. Eating happens less frequently.	Be sure to eat high fat with low carbs. Your body uses the fat to restore your fat built hormones. Elevated insulin within your body prevents you from using the stored fat. You must eat the fat.	
	#3: I "accidentally" missed a meal. [Keto-adapted]			Fat supplies the resources needed to make fat-built hormones approach healthy levels. Appetite decreases according to body's chemistry.	Sometimes it takes 10 weeks before this moment happens. Don't look at the scale. Listen for absence of hunger.	
	#4: Eat 2 meals per day	YOU DO THE WORK. Discipline needed for each new step.		Choose to eat only 2 meals per day.	Succeed 7 days in a row before advancing.	
BASELINE METABOLISM	**#5:** 16:8			Eat ALL food, snacks and supplements in an 8-hour window. No eating, snacking or chewing for 16 hours.	That means no gum during fasting hours. Suck on salt if you need a substitute. Keep your coffee filled with fat.	LIVE HERE
	#6: Advanced 16:8			Clean up your morning drink. Remove all calories and sweeteners. Morning drink = no fat, no MCT, no butter, no sweeteners, no calories. The 16 hours = only salt, water, black coffee or tea.	Don't remove the fat from your morning drink before this phase. You needed it to get here. Now it's time to let it go.	
	#7: 23:1 OMAD ALL in one hour			ALL calories and sweeteners in one hour. 23 hours = Only salt, water, tea or coffee.	Begin checking blood numbers right before you eat.	
	#8: Advanced 23:1/OMAD			Move eating-hour within 11 hours following sunrise to match your circadian rhythm.	Record the Dr. Boz ratio first thing in the morning. Repeat before eating.	
STRESSING METABOLISM	**#9:** 36-hour fast	PSYCHOLOGY. Use tribe for best results.	Blood Ketone Strips	Fast for 36 hours. No calories. No sweeteners. Start in evening as to use 2 cycles of sleep during the 36 hours.	Begin fast after evening meal. DANGER: If on blood pressure meds or blood sugar lowing meds. ASK YOUR DOCTOR.	USE INTERMITTENTLY
	#10: 36-hour fast without a celebration meal			After 36-hour fast, return to your normal pattern of eating without a splurge meal.	Offer a group fasting routine to others in your tribe. Fast together.	
	#11: 48-hour fast			Fast for 48 hours. No calories. No sweeteners.	Safe to try twice a week. Unlike the 36-hour fast, this option keeps meals at the same time each day.	
	#12: 72-hour fast			Fast for 72 hours. No calories. No sweeteners.	When the timing is right, stress your metabolism with 8 weeks of a 72-hour fast. The rest of the week, return to your BASELINE METABOLISM. The best transitions happen through this challenge.	

ketoCONTINUUM **Workbook**

ketoCONTINUUM Check-In Cards

#1 I eat every 2–4 hours	#7 23:1 OMAD: ALL in one hour. 23 hours=No calories or sweeteners.
#2 LESS THAN 20 total carbs. I eat every 6–8 hours.	#8 Advanced 23:1/OMAD. Your 1 hour of eating happens within the 11 hours following sunrise.
#3 I "accidentally" missed a meal. [Keto-adapted]	
#4 Eat 2 meals per day.	#9 36-hour fast
#5 16:8 ALL food, snacks, and supplements in an 8-hour window.	#10 36-hour fast without a celebration meal
#6 Advanced 16:8 Clean up morning drink. No calories or sweetener in AM drink.	#11 48-hour fast
	#12 72-hour fast

#1 I eat every 2–4 hours	#7 23:1 OMAD: ALL in one hour. 23 hours=No calories or sweeteners.
#2 LESS THAN 20 total carbs. I eat every 6–8 hours.	#8 Advanced 23:1/OMAD. Your 1 hour of eating happens within the 11 hours following sunrise.
#3 I "accidentally" missed a meal. [Keto-adapted]	
#4 Eat 2 meals per day.	#9 36-hour fast
#5 16:8 ALL food, snacks, and supplements in an 8-hour window.	#10 36-hour fast without a celebration meal
#6 Advanced 16:8 Clean up morning drink. No calories or sweetener in AM drink.	#11 48-hour fast
	#12 72-hour fast

#1 I eat every 2–4 hours	#7 23:1 OMAD: ALL in one hour. 23 hours=No calories or sweeteners.
#2 LESS THAN 20 total carbs. I eat every 6–8 hours.	#8 Advanced 23:1/OMAD. Your 1 hour of eating happens within the 11 hours following sunrise.
#3 I "accidentally" missed a meal. [Keto-adapted]	
#4 Eat 2 meals per day.	#9 36-hour fast
#5 16:8 ALL food, snacks, and supplements in an 8-hour window.	#10 36-hour fast without a celebration meal
#6 Advanced 16:8 Clean up morning drink. No calories or sweetener in AM drink.	#11 48-hour fast
	#12 72-hour fast

Time of last carb-meal
:

TIME	FOOD	TOTAL CARBS	HOW DO YOU FEEL?
8:00 am	Hard Boiled Eggs 6	26	Full

TOTAL CARBS =

DAY 2 CHART

DAY 2 DATE	TIME	BLOOD PRESSURE	HEART RATE	PEETONE STRIP COLOR	TOTAL CARBS	BOWEL ACTIVITY
				0 1 2 3 4 5 6		
				0 1 2 3 4 5 6		
				0 1 2 3 4 5 6		
				0 1 2 3 4 5 6		
				0 1 2 3 4 5 6		
				0 1 2 3 4 5 6		
				0 1 2 3 4 5 6		
				0 1 2 3 4 5 6		
				0 1 2 3 4 5 6		
				0 1 2 3 4 5 6		
				0 1 2 3 4 5 6		
				0 1 2 3 4 5 6		
				0 1 2 3 4 5 6		
				0 1 2 3 4 5 6		
				0 1 2 3 4 5 6		
				0 1 2 3 4 5 6		
				0 1 2 3 4 5 6		
				0 1 2 3 4 5 6		
				3 4 5 6		
				3 4 5 6		
				3 4 5 6		

DAY 3 CHART

DAY 3 DATE	TIME	BLOOD PRESSURE	HEART RATE	PEETONE STRIP COLOR	TOTAL CARBS	BOWEL ACTIVITY
				0 1 2 3 4 5 6		
				0 1 2 3 4 5 6		
				0 1 2 3 4 5 6		
				0 1 2 3 4 5 6		
				0 1 2 3 4 5 6		
				0 1 2 3 4 5 6		
				0 1 2 3 4 5 6		
				0 1 2 3 4 5 6		
				0 1 2 3 4 5 6		
				0 1 2 3 4 5 6		
				0 1 2 3 4 5 6		
				0 1 2 3 4 5 6		
				0 1 2 3 4 5 6		
				0 1 2 3 4 5 6		
				0 1 2 3 4 5 6		
				0 1 2 3 4 5 6		
				0 1 2 3 4 5 6		
				0 1 2 3 4 5 6		
				0 1 2 3 4 5		
				0 1 2 3 4 5		

ketoCONTINUUM Workbook

DAY 4 CHART

DAY 4 DATE	TIME	BLOOD PRESSURE	HEART RATE	PEETONE STRIP COLOR	TOTAL CARBS	BOWEL ACTIVITY
				0 1 2 3 4 5 6		
				0 1 2 3 4 5 6		
				0 1 2 3 4 5 6		
				0 1 2 3 4 5 6		
				0 1 2 3 4 5 6		
				0 1 2 3 4 5 6		
				0 1 2 3 4 5 6		
				0 1 2 3 4 5 6		
				0 1 2 3 4 5 6		
				0 1 2 3 4 5 6		
				0 1 2 3 4 5 6		
				0 1 2 3 4 5 6		
				0 1 2 3 4 5 6		
				0 1 2 3 4 5 6		
				0 1 2 3 4 5 6		
				0 1 2 3 4 5 6		
				0 1 2 3 4 5 6		
				0 1 2 3 4 5 6		
				0 1 2 3 4 5 6		
				0 1 2 3 4 5 6		

CHIA SEED CHARTS

CHIA SEEDS FOR BOWELS TOO SLOW: TAPER ON

Date	1 Tbsp	1 Tbsp	1 Tbsp	1 Tbsp	1 Tbsp	1 Tbsp	1 Tbsp	1 Tbsp	1 Tbsp	1 Tbsp	1 Tbsp	1 Tbsp
	Dose 1	Dose 2	Dose 3	Dose 4	Dose 5	Dose 6	Dose 7	Dose 8	Dose 9	Dose 10	Dose 11	Dose 12
Time												
	Dose 13	Dose 14	Dose 15	Dose 16	Dose 17	Dose 18	Dose 19	Dose 20	Dose 21	Dose 22	Dose 23	Dose 24
Time												

CHIA SEEDS TAPER OFF

Day of Protocol	Morning Dose	Noon Dose	Bowel movement?		Notes
Day 1	7 Tbsp	7 Tbsp	Yes / No		
Day 2	7 Tbsp	6 Tbsp	Yes / No		
Day 3	6 Tbsp	6 Tbsp	Yes / No		
Day 4	6 Tbsp	5 Tbsp	Yes / No		
Day 5	5 Tbsp	5 Tbsp	Yes / No		
Day 6	5 Tbsp	4 Tbsp	Yes / No		
Day 7	4 Tbsp	4 Tbsp	Yes / No		
Day 8	4 Tbsp	3 Tbsp	Yes / No		
Day 9	3 Tbsp	3 Tbsp	Yes / No		
Day 10	3 Tbsp	2 Tbsp	Yes / No		
Day 11	2 Tbsp	2 Tbsp	Yes / No		
Day 12	2 Tbsp	1 Tbsp	Yes / No		
Day 13	2 Tbsp		Yes / No		
Day 14	1 Tbsp		Yes / No		

ketoCONTINUUM Workbook

Date	Chia Seeds for Bowels Too Fast: Taper ON									
	1 TBSP	2 TBSPs	3 TBSPs	4 TBSPs	5 TBSPs	6 TBSPs	7 TBSPs	8 TBSPs	9 TBSPs	10 TBSPs
	loose stool 1	loose stool 2	loose stool 3	loose stool 4	loose stool 5	loose stool 6	loose stool 7	loose stool 8	loose stool 9	loose stool 10
Total number TBSPs of chia seeds	1 total	3 total	6 total	10 total	15 total	21 total	28 total	36 total	45 total	55 total

DAY 5 CHART

TIME	BLOOD PRESSURE	HEART RATE	PEETONE STRIP COLOR	TOTAL CARBS	BOWEL ACTIVITY
			0 1 2 3 4 5 6		
			0 1 2 3 4 5 6		
			0 1 2 3 4 5 6		
			0 1 2 3 4 5 6		
			0 1 2 3 4 5 6		
			0 1 2 3 4 5 6		
			0 1 2 3 4 5 6		
			0 1 2 3 4 5 6		
			0 1 2 3 4 5 6		
			0 1 2 3 4 5 6		
			0 1 2 3 4 5 6		
			0 1 2 3 4 5 6		
			0 1 2 3 4 5 6		
			0 1 2 3 4 5 6		
			0 1 2 3 4 5 6		
			0 1 2 3 4 5 6		
			0 1 2 3 4 5 6		

ketoCONTINUUM Workbook

MAGNESIUM SHORTAGE SYMPTOMS CHART

	Week 1	Week 2	Week 3
# Magnesium Soaks/Baths in Past Week	1 2 3 4 5 6 7	1 2 3 4 5 6 7	1 2 3 4 5 6 7
Days You Swallowed Magnesium Supplements	1 2 3 4 5 6 7	1 2 3 4 5 6 7	1 2 3 4 5 6 7
Energy	HIGH Medium Low	HIGH Medium Low	HIGH Medium Low
Concentration	FOCUSED Distracted	FOCUSED Distracted	FOCUSED Distracted
Motivation	MOTIVATED Unmotivated	MOTIVATED Unmotivated	MOTIVATED Unmotivated
Days of Bowel Movement	1 2 3 4 5 6 7	1 2 3 4 5 6 7	1 2 3 4 5 6 7
Muscle Cramps	NO CRAMPS Cramps	NO CRAMPS Cramps	NO CRAMPS Cramps
Headaches	NO PAIN Headaches	NO PAIN Headaches	NO PAIN Headaches
Back Pain (muscle)	NO PAIN Back Pain	NO PAIN Back Pain	NO PAIN Back Pain
Neck Pain (muscle)	NO PAIN Neck Pain	NO PAIN Neck Pain	NO PAIN Neck Pain
Tremor	NO TREMOR Trembling	NO TREMOR Trembling	NO TREMOR Trembling
Mood (Depression)	NONE Depressed	NONE Depressed	NONE Depressed
Mood (Worried)	NONE Worried	NONE Worried	NONE Worried
Memory	NORMAL Forgetful	NORMAL Forgetful	NORMAL Forgetful
Brain Fog	NONE Foggy	NONE Foggy	NONE Foggy
Mood (Grouchy)	NONE Grouchy	NONE Grouchy	NONE Grouchy

DAY 6 CHART

TIME	BLOOD PRESSURE	HEART RATE	PEETONE STRIP COLOR	TOTAL CARBS	BOWEL ACTIVITY
			0 1 2 3 4 5 6		
			0 1 2 3 4 5 6		
			0 1 2 3 4 5 6		
			0 1 2 3 4 5 6		
			0 1 2 3 4 5 6		
			0 1 2 3 4 5 6		
			0 1 2 3 4 5 6		
			0 1 2 3 4 5 6		
			0 1 2 3 4 5 6		
			0 1 2 3 4 5 6		
			0 1 2 3 4 5 6		
			0 1 2 3 4 5 6		
			0 1 2 3 4 5 6		
			0 1 2 3 4 5 6		
			0 1 2 3 4 5 6		
			0 1 2 3 4 5 6		
			0 1 2 3 4 5 6		
			0 1 2 3 4 5 6		

ketoCONTINUUM Workbook

FOOD CRAVING SUMMARY CHART

Date	What time of day did it happen?	Emotions Associated		How long did the sensation last?		What made it go away?	
		CRAVING	HUNGER	CRAVING	HUNGER	CRAVING	HUNGER
		YES	NO	<5 MIN	>15 MIN	• Meditation singing • Splash water to your face • Salt to your tongue • Go for a walk	Time
		YES	NO	<5 MIN	>15 MIN		Time
		YES	NO	<5 MIN	>15 MIN		Time
		YES	NO	<5 MIN	>15 MIN		Time
		YES	NO	<5 MIN	>15 MIN		Time
		YES	NO	<5 MIN	>15 MIN		Time
		YES	NO	<5 MIN	>15 MIN		Time
		YES	NO	<5 MIN	>15 MIN		Time
		YES	NO	<5 MIN	>15 MIN		Time
		YES	NO	<5 MIN	>15 MIN		Time

10-MINUTE FOOD CRAVING EXERCISE

Which food are you craving?								
Date	Time	Salt Crystal	Desire Level					Notes: What else is on your mind? What is going on around you? Which emotion do you feel?
	Start	Yes / No	1	2	3	4	5	
	0:30 sec	Yes / No	1	2	3	4	5	
	1:00	Yes / No	1	2	3	4	5	
	1:30	Yes / No	1	2	3	4	5	
	2:00	Yes / No	1	2	3	4	5	
	2:30	Yes / No	1	2	3	4	5	
	3:00	Yes / No	1	2	3	4	5	
	3:30	Yes / No	1	2	3	4	5	
	4:00	Yes / No	1	2	3	4	5	
	4:30	Yes / No	1	2	3	4	5	
	5:00	Yes / No	1	2	3	4	5	
	5:30	Yes / No	1	2	3	4	5	
	6:00	Yes / No	1	2	3	4	5	
	6:30	Yes / No	1	2	3	4	5	
	7:00	Yes / No	1	2	3	4	5	
	7:30	Yes / No	1	2	3	4	5	
	8:00	Yes / No	1	2	3	4	5	
	8:30	Yes / No	1	2	3	4	5	
	9:00	Yes / No	1	2	3	4	5	
	9:30	Yes / No	1	2	3	4	5	
	10:00	Yes / No	1	2	3	4	5	

ketoCONTINUUM Workbook

10-MINUTE FOOD CRAVING EXERCISE

Which food are you craving?

Date	Time	Salt Crystal	Desire Level					Notes: What else is on your mind? What is going on around you? Which emotion do you feel?
	Start	Yes / No	1	2	3	4	5	
	0:30 sec	Yes / No	1	2	3	4	5	
	1:00	Yes / No	1	2	3	4	5	
	1:30	Yes / No	1	2	3	4	5	
	2:00	Yes / No	1	2	3	4	5	
	2:30	Yes / No	1	2	3	4	5	
	3:00	Yes / No	1	2	3	4	5	
	3:30	Yes / No	1	2	3	4	5	
	4:00	Yes / No	1	2	3	4	5	
	4:30	Yes / No	1	2	3	4	5	
	5:00	Yes / No	1	2	3	4	5	
	5:30	Yes / No	1	2	3	4	5	
	6:00	Yes / No	1	2	3	4	5	
	6:30	Yes / No	1	2	3	4	5	
	7:00	Yes / No	1	2	3	4	5	
	7:30	Yes / No	1	2	3	4	5	
	8:00	Yes / No	1	2	3	4	5	
	8:30	Yes / No	1	2	3	4	5	
	9:00	Yes / No	1	2	3	4	5	
	9:30	Yes / No	1	2	3	4	5	
	10:00	Yes / No	1	2	3	4	5	

CHALLENGES CHART

Day: Challenge	1st Success	
DAY 8: Consume only calorie-free unsweetened drinks.		
DAY 9: Eat a can of sardines.		
DAY 10: Identify your accountability partner.		
DAY 11: Take a magnesium bath or float.		
DAY 12: Conduct a craving analysis exercise. [Chart found in Section 2.8]		
DAY 13: Watch the sleep lecture. Fill out the sleep chart.		
DAY 14: Test your social strength.		

ketoCONTINUUM Workbook

2nd Success	3rd Success	4th Success

WEEK 2 CHART

Date	Time	Blood Pressure	Heart Rate	PeeTone Strip Color	Total Carbs	Bowel Activity	Challenge Completed
				0 1 2 3 4 5 6			
				0 1 2 3 4 5 6			
				0 1 2 3 4 5 6			
				0 1 2 3 4 5 6			
				0 1 2 3 4 5 6			
				0 1 2 3 4 5 6			
				0 1 2 3 4 5 6			
				0 1 2 3 4 5 6			
				0 1 2 3 4 5 6			
				0 1 2 3 4 5 6			
				0 1 2 3 4 5 6			
				0 1 2 3 4 5 6			
				0 1 2 3 4 5 6			
				0 1 2 3 4 5 6			
				0 1 2 3 4 5 6			

ketoCONTINUUM Workbook

KETO**CONTINUUM #3**

WEEK 5	Day 1	Day 2	Day 3	Day 4	Day 5	Day 6	Day 7
Blood Pressure							
PeeTones							
Symptoms of Low Magnesium							
Epsom Salt Bath/Float							
Accountability Partner Check-in							
Number of Unsweetened Drinks							
Meal 1 Time							
Meal 2 Time							
Meal 3 Time							
I accidentally missed a meal							
Hours Slept							
Weight							

KETO**CONTINUUM #4**

WEEK __	Day 1	Day 2	Day 3	Day 4	Day 5	Day 6	Day 7
Blood Pressure							
PeeTones							
Symptoms of Low Magnesium							
Epsom Salt Bath/Float							
Accountability Partner Check-in							
Number of Unsweetened Drinks							
Meal 1 Time							
Meal 2 Time							
Consecutive Days of 2 Meals Per Day	1 2 3 4 5 6 7	1 2 3 4 5 6 7	1 2 3 4 5 6 7	1 2 3 4 5 6 7	1 2 3 4 5 6 7	1 2 3 4 5 6 7	1 2 3 4 5 6 7
Hours Slept							
Exercise							
Weight (Only once/ week)							

keto**CONTINUUM #5**

Date	TIME: First Bite	TIME: Last Bite	Did you keep the food within 8 hours?	How many days in a row did you keep to 8 hours of consumption?	# of drinks with calories or sweeteners
			Yes/No 1 4 8 12 16	1 2 3 4 5 6 7	
			Yes/No 1 4 8 12 16	1 2 3 4 5 6 7	
			Yes/No 1 4 8 12 16	1 2 3 4 5 6 7	
			Yes/No 1 4 8 12 16	1 2 3 4 5 6 7	
			Yes/No 1 4 8 12 16	1 2 3 4 5 6 7	
			Yes/No 1 4 8 12 16	1 2 3 4 5 6 7	
			Yes/No 1 4 8 12 16	1 2 3 4 5 6 7	
			Yes/No 1 4 8 12 16	1 2 3 4 5 6 7	
			Yes/No 1 4 8 12 16	1 2 3 4 5 6 7	
			Yes/No 1 4 8 12 16	1 2 3 4 5 6 7	
			Yes/No 1 4 8 12 16	1 2 3 4 5 6 7	

DR. BOZ RATIO CHART

Date:	Time of Measurement	# Hours Fasting	Glucose mg/dL	Glucose mmol/L	Ketone mmol/L	Glucose:Ketone Index	Dr. Boz Ratio	Minutes of Exercise/Sauna	Blood Pressure

Heart Rate	Weight (limit to weekly)	Total Hours Slept	Total Carbs Protein Grams	Meal Time(s) / Notes

ketoCONTINUUM #6

Date	TIME: First Bite or Sip (first calorie or sweeteners)		When you will stop all calories, chewing and sweeteners	How many days in a row did you make it?
		Add 8 hours >		1 2 3 4 5 6 7
		Add 8 hours >		1 2 3 4 5 6 7
		Add 8 hours >		1 2 3 4 5 6 7
		Add 8 hours >		1 2 3 4 5 6 7
		Add 8 hours >		1 2 3 4 5 6 7
		Add 8 hours >		1 2 3 4 5 6 7
		Add 8 hours >		1 2 3 4 5 6 7
		Add 8 hours >		1 2 3 4 5 6 7
		Add 8 hours >		1 2 3 4 5 6 7
		Add 8 hours >		1 2 3 4 5 6 7
		Add 8 hours >		1 2 3 4 5 6 7

ketoCONTINUUM Workbook

ketoCONTINUUM #7

	Wake Up Time	Morning STATS (Measure at routine times)			GOAL: Keep eating within the hours from 6 AM to 11 PM		GOAL: Reduce # of hours
		Glucose	Ketones	Dr. Boz Ratio	Eating Window Time Open	Eating Window Time Closed	# of Hours for Eating Window
WEEK ___							
SUN							1 4 8
MON							1 4 8
TUE							1 4 8
WED							1 4 8
THU							1 4 8
FRI							1 4 8
SAT							1 4 8
WEEK ___							
SUN							1 4 8
MON							1 4 8
TUE							1 4 8
WED							1 4 8
THU							1 4 8
FRI							1 4 8
SAT							1 4 8

KETOCONTINUUM #8-#12

	Morning STATS (Measure at routine time)			Break-Fast STATS (Measure right before eating/ drinking your first calorie)			TIME: Last Bite / Calorie	TIME: First Bite/ Calorie that Broke the Fast	Total Hours Fasted
	Glucose	Ketones	Dr. Boz Ratio	Break-Fast Glucose	Break-Fast Ketones	Break-Fast Dr Boz Ratio			
WEEK ____									
SUN									
MON									
TUE									
WED									
THU									
FRI									
SAT									
WEEK ____									
SUN									
MON									
TUES									
WED									
THU									
FRI									
SAT									

ketoCONTINUUM Workbook

														GOAL: Resume Your Standard Window
							GOAL: Find a rhythm for fasting. Track your numbers. Watch for patterns that lead to success and those that predict a stumble.								
6-7 AM	8 AM	9 AM	10-11 AM	12 Noon	1-2 PM	3-4 PM	5 PM	6 PM	7 PM	8 PM	9 PM	10 PM	11-12 Mid night	1-5 AM	# of Hours for Eating Window
															1 4 8
															1 4 8
															1 4 8
															1 4 8
															1 4 8
															1 4 8
															1 4 8
															1 4 8
															1 4 8
															1 4 8
															1 4 8
															1 4 8
															1 4 8
															1 4 8

ketoCONTINUUM Workbook

ketoCONTINUUM Workbook